This book, by taking psycholog.   day,
formulates a diet, that by being more varied and sensual, tackles the gluttony
and excess that is facilitated by our consumerist society. By heightening the
pleasures gained from both food and sex, rather than temporarily losing
weight shrouded in an atmosphere of denial, this diet is sustainable. Herbs
play an essential culinary role, but their capacity to enhance both sexual
performance and pleasure is always close at hand.

To the
Happy 75th
Birthday

Jun

Herb and Sex Diet

Simon Taylor

S J Taylor

SJT

Herb and Sex Diet
Copyright © 2006 Simon Taylor

First published in Great Britain

S J Taylor
http://myweb.tiscali.co.uk/herbandsexdiet

ISBN 978-0-9553954-0-6

Illustrations: Simon Taylor
Designer: Simon Taylor

Printed by Lightning Source UK Ltd

To Alison

Contents

Why?

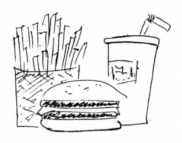

Introduction

Why?

It goes without saying that food has a central place in our lives. It has had a pivotal position in many of our celebrations and always has done. Feast days are a feature of all human societies. Food is used to entertain and impress throughout society, from individuals to governments courting visiting dignitaries. We watch multiple television programmes and flick through endless pages of Sunday supplements about food. Huge swathes of industry depend on packaging and repackaging food. We have food writers, photographers and critics. For sufferers of eating disorders it takes on a more malign role, eating (or often not eating) becoming an expression of distress or entrapment. For all of us foods become associated with particular events in our lives, individual foods becoming imbued with emotional salience. Most of all, however, food is one of life's great pleasures; a pleasure that can and should be enjoyed with each meal. This idea does not hold a central position in the British psyche as it does for the French, who do not regard the enjoyment of good food as the domain only of the privileged. With the rise of fast food, however, even the Gallic kings of gastronomy are fearful that their heritage will be lost. My passion for good food has been derided by my peers but in retrospect maybe bordered on the obsessional. For example, I took the BSE crisis in the late eighties (the science about which for a time was so blurred that it seemed conceivable that any farmed animal was a potential risk) to indulge my love of game. Indeed this was the only meat I ate for about two years and marvellous it was too.

Three years ago I was told that I had high blood pressure. Hypertension is often a sign of being overweight and physically unfit. It is in fact usually symptomless but can lead to a myriad of health problems including heart attacks, strokes and impotence. Drug treatments for raised blood pressure are not without side effects, impotence not being uncommon. This then posed to me a dual threat. Not only was I to cut down on my eating but potential problems were posed to my sex life. Was I to be denied the indulgence of the two greatest pleasures in life? Oh hell on earth!

I had always been fat, attracting the nickname of Tubby from the tender age of seven. My previous attempts to lose weight had failed dreadfully and problems worsened as failures accumulated. There was an incremental increase of my waist size after the failure of each diet. This was attributed by some of my biological relatives to "fat genes". At the time there was a rising tide of public health concern about obesity. The problem seemed more acute in the USA. Did Americans have more fat genes than the British? This explanation seemed unlikely. I was facing a dilemma; I had to lose weight but I had a busy professional job and the potential stress of denying myself food, or at least certain foods, I saw as a stress too far. The last straw to break the camel's back. Denial had always failed before and there was no way I was going to fill in diaries or be weighed in front of a group of strangers. I had to do something and I had to start right now!

I have always been fascinated by why people do what they do. Observing people, particularly in spaces where we wait, leads to speculation and wonder about the narratives of their lives. Who is the chap on the train who looks like a tramp and yet reads the Times Literary Supplement? Why does the guy at the airport roll his cigarette so precisely but repeatedly that most of the tobacco falls out? What has brought them to these places and where are they going? Not surprisingly then, the fascination with my young son went beyond that of paternal love. Until his first burger and chips from a fast food outlet he had happily tucked into whatever we were eating whether this be *coq au vin* and new potatoes or pheasant on white cabbage cooked in white wine with juniper. After one fast food meal it was as if his palate had been transformed and it is only now, after ten years, that his tastes are beginning to widen again. I may be paranoid, but I sniffed a sense of conspiracy. Could it be that our tastes and diet are being influenced and manipulated? And if so by whom?

I cannot remember the gestation period, but this diet was born out of an eclectic mix of ideas borrowed from many areas. These included evolution theory, psychology (in particular motivation theories and my own academic research project about sexual motivation), cognitive therapy and ecological epidemiology. Herbs play an important role in this diet not only for their culinary use but also perhaps, more peripheral to mainstream science, there is also a sprinkling of ideas from herbalism. Although often dismissed, there is certainly evidence that a small number of these treatments work; perhaps the most thoroughly researched being St John's Wort and mild depression. Sex and sensuality are also important ingredients in this diet, and given the claims of the aphrodisiac properties of various herbs, I am sure that I am not alone in being tantalised by the idea that one or more of these is some natural form of Viagra that will enhance our sexual pleasure and performance.

Most importantly this diet had to square the circle of my love for food and the need to diet, a problem that faces many. In the chapters that follow I try to give an account of a theoretical basis for the possible causes of obesity in our modern age and why other diets may not succeed. Given this insight I suggest how we can individually lose weight more successfully while still having fun. I have included a number of recipes that I have found enjoyable and helpful, and these should stimulate your own exploration of cuisine.

I am not a nutritionalist and as a result calorie counts do not appear. The recipes encourage the use of a variety of fresh ingredients, which should ensure adequate vitamins, minerals and essential oils. Although dieting during pregnancy is strongly not recommended, if you are pregnant and your partner wishes to commence this diet (which involves more than usual amounts of herbs) you would be advised to consult a dietician or a qualified herbalist.

Thoughts

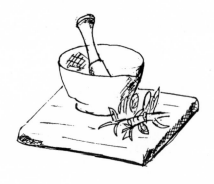

Chapter 1

Thoughts

CYCLES

Many people diet either on one regime or another. These diets seem to come and go as quickly as hairstyles, skirt lengths or mobile phones. Legendary diets however do not seem to find that metaphorical crock of gold at the end of the rainbow. Why then do so many diets fail, and since masochism is not a common human trait, why do we keep returning for more?

There are many traps for those who are overweight and try to lose their excess. Although it is obvious that feeling hungry on a diet can make it difficult to stick to, there are problems that go beyond this. Indeed there seem to be several unhelpful cycles; what we might call "cycles of demoralisation". These are vicious cycles, which potentially undermine our motivation by affecting our mood, relationships and resolve. An example of this is how being on a diet makes us feel. Usually, the diet is viewed as a problem and makes us feel stressed. There is a tendency then to face other of life's problems negatively or pessimistically. As a result we feel unhappy and irritable. This in itself may be enough to give up our commitment to continue to diet, or it may highlight other existing difficulties in our lives. These may be at work or may be in some aspect of our relationships. A missed deadline or a partner's comment about being less communicative since the diet started may be the last straw and out come the crisps, cream buns and chocolate. Problems seem to get on top of us more and comfort eating may in itself be used as the mechanism to cope.

Obesity may also lead to unfitness, health problems and potentially unattractiveness to your partner. Your sex life may suffer. I have clear memories of being told to "Get off, you're too heavy" and "You're squashing me". Although such negative comments may be partly aimed at encouragement to lose weight, they all too often add to a sense of demoralisation and potential resentment. This may be particularly so if you are trying to diet and have already deprived yourself of two or three of your favourite nibbles that day. Rather than being encouraging the effect may well be to make you give up altogether.

Many diets also have strict rules; so many points a day, no cheese, no chocolate or mayonnaise. It is true that we all live by rules, without which society would crumble, but not all rules have equal weight and the consequences of breaking them are not equal either. Committing murder or indulging in a particularly mature Lincolnshire Poacher cheese do not equate although sometimes we react almost as if they do. Denial and guilt are intimate bedfellows, and guilt, like other negative emotions, is akin to punishment and therefore tends to be a poor long-term motivator. Should the threat of feeling like a bad person hang over you all the time while you are

15

dieting? The main problems here are that not only do you feel dysphoric but you have set up a situation that can quickly facilitate the end of your dieting. If you transgress once or twice then what is the point of continuing to stick to the rules? You may as well be hung for a sheep as a lamb!

The other major trap is that if you have managed to negotiate problems so far and get *the courgette and bran diet* to work it is unwise to take all your size sixteen dresses to the charity shop and go on an extensive shopping spree for those *Olympic gold* size twelves. Just for how long can you just eat courgettes and bran? How healthy is it? And to what expense to the quality of your life? After all, didn't you used to enjoy food? Maintenance and sustainability are key to continued success. Whether you can maintain your weight depends partly on why you wanted to lose weight in the first place and partly whether the changes you have made have been worth it. If you have been able to lose weight and also feel that there are other tangible benefits, the balance will be in favour of maintenance.

The words "dieting" and "pleasure" are seldom found in the same sentence. This diet attempts to be different by improving your cuisine and hopefully your sex life. It sets in train cycles of change (heightening your appreciation and pleasure of and passion for life) that are sustainable.

MOTIVES

There are almost daily reports in the media that we are becoming an unfit and overweight population placing many of us at significant risk of health problems including diabetes, high blood pressure, heart disease and strokes. Despite this knowledge we continue to eat too much. We are, of course, all free individuals which is why we become increasingly irritated by the *food police* issuing what appear to be an ever-increasing flood of pronouncements about what we should and shouldn't eat. We all have free will and if we want to eat too much of this or that (but especially cream buns and salty chips) then it is up to us and blow the consequences.

I suspect it is not an uncommon experience (particularly after an evening out) to reflect that, "Although that was a great meal, I feel bloated, I need a rest before lying down and going to bed". We feel uncomfortable, we know we have eaten too much but we really wanted the sautéed potatoes and then the toffee pudding and the cream. We know there are consequences, indigestion for one and as for sex that is off the menu completely now! And we know that our trousers will feel even tighter tomorrow morning.

So why then don't we learn? Are all overweight people stupid? Why do we eat so much, and why is it that it is the high calorie foods we overdo? This raises the question about whether we genuinely do exercise free will in the way we eat? Attempting to answer to these questions may put us in a better position to master the problem of overeating and help us change our eating habits.

Firstly, I presume that having purchased or borrowed this book you feel that you have a problem with being overweight. Acknowledgement of this is necessary before you can do anything about it. All too often this recognition is only sufficient to swing us into all but temporary action. A New Year's resolution, "I'll lose weight for the summer holiday" or " I gave up after the weekend away last year but I'll stick to it this year". But what happened last year? You had lost six pounds over the previous month; it was not a bad diet, the banning of chocolate seemed harsh, but evidently it had been working. Yes you had been under stress, a poor appraisal at work the week before and that presentation had gone badly despite staying up half the night to complete it. And who would blame you (except yourself!) for trying the chef's famous speciality chocolate mousse? Sometimes it may seem that the whole process of dieting is a pointless waste of time. You start, you give up, you need larger trousers again! "What was the point of that? I'll try again next year."

Stop a moment. Take a step back and ask yourself, "Why am I dieting?" The answers vary. Happiness? "If I was not so fat I would have a better time?" Success? "If I was thinner then I would be more successful at work?" Confidence? "My obesity makes me feel self conscious." Or are you doing it for someone else? Clarity in your own understanding as to why you are embarking on a diet is a key to success. Your diet will not make you a better person. It will not resolve relationship or work problems. It will not make you more popular or the life and soul of the party, and it will probably have no effect on your self-esteem.

In addition to the *why* question you also need to ask do you really want to diet *now*? Well, would it make any difference? What if you don't bother? You could put the book back on the shelf and just leave the shop. Or if it was a present, take it back, say it was a duplicate, and you haven't opened this copy. At this stage it may not be a bad idea to draw up a pros and cons list. Some people find it helpful to draw this up as a simple matrix, with the columns as *pros* and *cons* and the rows as *Dieting now* and *Changing nothing at the moment*. Clearly there will be some repetition, with pros for dieting also appearing as cons for doing nothing.

You may also find that on the cons side for dieting may be the argument that you enjoy food too much and this is where this book may help. As I have said, I am passionate about food. The pleasures of eating are some of the greatest in life. I'll quite happily drive miles to a good restaurant or to buy some brilliant traditional cheese. I hope that as a result of this diet, rather than your pleasure being diminished by restrictions, it will be enhanced and your love of food revitalized.

Almost as important as the *why* and *why now* questions is whether you will know when you have reached your target or indeed do you have one? It is important that it is achievable and realistic. It is easier to have a goal that is more objective than a vague statement like "looking slim". Setting a weight or dress size is far better but ensure that it is reasonable. If you are in the top five percent of the population with regard to your weight at the moment then to aim to be in the bottom five percent would be unrealistic and potentially unhealthy. If you are in the top five percent then perhaps you do have a tendency to be heavier than average and aiming for a weight a bit above average would be more reasonable. For me it was not a particular waist size or weight, but to normalise my blood pressure. Perhaps having a health goal was easier but certainly aiming for a particular body shape is more difficult and potentially unhelpful. It is important to remember that over the centuries what has been regarded as attractive in the human form has changed. We should not compare ourselves negatively with the beautiful human forms portrayed in advertisements around us. Their contemporary perfection actually turns them into freaks.

So having given the decision due consideration and deciding that, not only do you want to lose weight now but you feel sufficiently committed to see it through, surely it is only a matter of remaining resolute. We just need enough will power? This brings us back to the question of whether we genuinely exercise free will in the choices of the way we eat. We are after all thinking animals and our basic instincts can be subservient to our intellect. When it comes to sex, activity in animals is determined directly or indirectly by hormonal status, whereas in us this is only a minor component. For us there are many factors, which interact including social norms, where we are, how we are thinking (which may include our fantasies) and how we feel. Intellectual processes also clearly do influence some of our choices of what we eat and drink; for example why else may we choose to spend thirteen pounds on a bottle of wine when it is possible to buy what is effectively the same stuff for ten pounds less. We are aware that our taste buds are there for more than checking whether something is poisonous or contains minerals that may be in short supply and our noses are there for more than the redundant task of finding our prey or a fertile mate. These sensory organs now enable us to savour taste and variety of flavour and help us make decisions based on the pleasure we derive from food and drink, or so we may think.

Hunger is a basic drive; we need to eat to survive. This certainly was a priority for our forbears. Those who ate a lot at times of plenty and who ate efficiently could stock up their energy reserves better. Not all that is edible has much energy. Green vegetables may be a source of some vitamins and roughage but contain little available energy. In an environment of uncertainty about food supply an appetite for high fat and sugar foods was an advantage. Accumulating fat reserves would help survival when food was

18

scarce although there may be a downside to this; reducing agility for hunting. We have, however, always lived in groups, and perhaps a small proportion of a tribe would be more energetic, adventurous and always looking for new things. They would find new hunting grounds or innovate or invent in other ways giving the tribe an edge in finding food. A tribe that contained a mixture of people with different predispositions would probably survive best and would have been at greatest evolutionary advantage. In our modern highly regulated western society these energetic adventurous people might run into problems and attract the label of attention deficit disorder. Similarly those who were more efficient at storing energy and who would have helped the tribe survive at times of famine would, in our society, in which we are fortunate that food is freely available, be those who may run into problems by being most likely to become obese.

This is not the whole story. Although it may explain why some people are more prone to becoming overweight, it does not explain why it seems that a greater and greater proportion of us are becoming obese. It is useful at this point to examine some of the factors that affect our appetite. We need to start with the idea that the body usually reacts to situations so as to maintain the status quo within itself. The biological term is homeostasis. Homeostasis allows the body to find a natural balance and keeps things steady. If we have been working on a hot day, we sweat and because we have lost water our body reacts so that we do not become dehydrated. Our kidneys produce less, but therefore more concentrated, urine and we feel thirsty and drink. We also sweat when hot to stop us from over-heating. Our bodies are in fact very good at keeping our body temperature level; this is why we shiver when we are cold so that our muscles can generate heat. This is like the thermostat in our houses or the climate control in our cars. Our bodies are full of these systems to keep things steady. It was once believed that our drive to eat (our appetite) was controlled in a similar way. This principle however does not seem to apply to our eating habits or indeed to sex. It is true that when our first line energy stores are running low, we feel hungry. We stock up by eating but we seem unable to stop when those energy stores are replaced. We have a second helping of trifle, another slice of Stilton or just one more wafer-thin mint. Often we only stop when we feel bloated. And it is usually the high-energy foods packed with sugar and fat that we continue to eat. These are the foods that give us the biggest kick; its almost as though they make us more hungry. They re-stimulate or excite our appetite to make us eat more almost like an addiction. How often have you been in two minds as to whether you could manage a sticky toffee pudding but could murder a second after the first or at least have no doubts about *petit-fours* or chocolates with coffee. This phenomenon is found in the rest of the animal kingdom too. Certainly, laboratory rats love cheese and chocolate bars and will grow excessively rotund if given free access to these; so rotund that they are virtually unable to move. It is the ability of these foods to stimulate appetite coupled with the change in the situation or environment with free availability of high stimulus foods that leads to this over eating. There are parallels here with salt, which seems to have a similar basic appetitive drive as sugar and fat. Salt, like energy, is an essential component of all our diets but it seems we cannot get enough. Testament to this is the central role it has played in many civilisations. It has been made into coinage and Roman legionnaires were paid in bags of salt, a *salarium*, from which the word salary is derived. In common with most essentials it has been the subject of taxation at some point in most countries. The swingeing rates that reached over 10,000% contributed to the start of the French revolution and Mahatma Gandhi's defiance of the iniquitous British salt taxes mobilised support for self-rule for India.

The conclusions that can be drawn from all this are that foods that are high in sugar, fat and salt actually stimulate our hunger and drive us to eat more and more of them. This would have been an advantage when food was potentially scarce; to make hay, as it were, while the sun was shining. We now live in an environment that is quite different with (at least for those in Western society) freely available food all the time. To compound the problem, so called "junk food" panders to these basic food drives and is indeed promoted with fast moving, colourful loud and exciting advertisements. It is no surprise then that children in particular will choose chips over boiled potatoes or chocolate over apples. Therefore, although some people may be at greater risk, we are all susceptible. With an increasing number of people being overweight, it seems that everyone runs the gauntlet of excess adipose tissue. It is only an awareness or insight into these once biologically advantageous drives and how they can be potentially exploited that can help us genuinely exercise free will and gain greater mastery in the way we choose what we eat.

PRINCIPLES

We have already discussed cycles of demoralisation and the traps caused by our survival instincts. Armed with this it may be possible to set in motion a new set of cycles; positive cycles.

First of all even if only one of you feels you need to lose weight this diet is a joint adventure. Your partner will by now know what you are doing. You will have to tell them about it. They will need to understand that occasionally you may be a little grumpy but also that there are many potential positives for both of you. For example, even before you get to the last chapter, the food that you eat will improve both in its quality and its variety. If you feel your partner is on board with your diet this will increase your own commitment especially if he or she can be encouraging. This is the first potential opportunity for positive feedback.

Secondly; rather than making you grumpy, this diet may have a direct positive effect on your mood. It is rich in vitamins, minerals and essential fatty acids, which have been shown to reduce irritability in clinical trials. In addition, surprisingly little but regular aerobic exercise lowers blood pressure, improves general fitness and lifts your mood. Why not defer dessert, set an earlier time to go to bed and make love later instead. Not only will you have missed probably the most calorie laden course, you will have used up some calories and taken at least that day's aerobic exercise. You may begin to feel healthier and invigorated rather than hungry; and instead of being grumpy you may find your spirits improve, a spring in your step and a smile on your face.

Guilt, as we have discussed, has potentially a malignant influence on dieting. This diet should not induce guilt, as it has no strict rules, calorie counting or diaries. It should actually reduce these feelings by encouraging you to try new things, any things, and experiment. Enjoying your food more, rather than feeling guilty, will become a further cycle for positive feedback. Sex, being a taboo-laden subject, is not uncommonly associated with some feelings of guilt as well. Despite living in a society in which sex seems to be thrust in our faces and there are regular reports of the sexual antics of celebrities and documentaries about wife swapping and group sex, many of us remain inhibited particularly with our partners about discussing our likes, dislikes and fantasies. Poor communication may also extend into other areas and generate resentment. However in an atmosphere of open, frank and consensual discussion about our own and our partner's sexual desires these feelings of guilt should be reduced. This is not only another opportunity for positive feedback, for example, a simple comment about how someone looks, or that sex is much more pleasurable now that they have lost some weight, but for development of your sexual relationship.

Lastly, but most of all, this diet will increase your appreciation of food and this increased passion may extend into other areas of your life. I have noticed that by cutting out a significant amount of sugar and fat I have become much more aware of subtle flavours. This increased appreciation of food will help maintain the changes you have achieved. Beyond this however, I would like to propose that a heightened pleasure in one area of one's life or modality can heighten the pleasure felt in others; a "synergistic aestheticism". This perhaps needs a little elaboration. We can certainly identify with the opposite, and have discussed it above, namely that when we are stressed and unhappy there is a tendency to be more pessimistic about other areas of our life and gain less pleasure from them. Perhaps the most overt and extreme example of synergistic aestheticism is when we fall in love. Usually the world looks brighter, opportunities appear wider and the world is generally a more joyous place. It is possible that by increasing your passion for, and enjoyment of food you may get more out of sex and vice versa. This could also positively affect other aspects of your life. What I hope to help you achieve with this diet is not only weight loss, but also a greater sense of sensuality and pleasure. Which comes first does not really matter. There are a few guiding principles that help negate the cycles of demoralisation, facilitate the positive cycles and therefore lay the foundations for enduring change.

Firstly, let me introduce you to what I call the "pleasure to calorie ratio" principle. This does indeed mean that you can eat anything. There are no banned foods. Instead you need to ask yourself two questions: is the pleasure worth the calories and how can I maximise on that pleasure? For example, chocolate has a truly unique and seductive flavour that in many people almost generates an insurmountable craving. Don't buy 250 grams of cheap chocolate from the newsagent when you buy a paper. You may have nibbled half of it before you even reach the crossword. Instead make a trip to a specialist shop, spend the same amount of money on a hundred grams of a high cocoa content Belgian and have it with your coffee once or twice a week, shared with your partner after a relaxing meal.

As you will see from the above example the second principle of "quality over quantity" is closely linked to the first idea. It is about maximising the experience rather than just refuelling. Again, pass over the twelve-ounce bargain steaks in the supermarket, spend the same amount on some well-hung fillet.

The third principle is that of "preparation". All the recipes in this book are time economic but require some effort, although in my own experience compared with the time required to serve up apparently "instant meals" the difference is small, and the term "instant" illusory. Preparation gives you a sense of control: yes you will be adding salt, but you know how much. But preparation goes beyond this; the aromas, the colours and the tactile feel of putting good food together is like foreplay generating an anticipation and tide of desire that increases the final pleasure. Food preparation, like foreplay, enhances both experiences respectively; they become more satisfying and there is no need to go back for something more. Although it goes without saying that you need to be in the mood for sex this is equally true when it comes to cooking. If you just don't feel like it, forget it and tell your partner. Ask them to cook, or just do something very simple. I would recommend the former since I think you can even make a hash of beans on toast if you just don't have your heart in it. You can however get yourself in the mood by thinking about your meal before getting home or even phoning or e-mailing your partner about it in the day. Ideally, sit down together with an aperitif and unwind, preferably next to the herb garden. This should inspire one of you.

Thoughts

"Variety" is the fourth principle. Variety itself is exciting and therefore heightens pleasure and can be motivating. The saying "a change is as good as a rest" seems to have validity. Variety and change can help you maintain the motivation that so often evaporates with other diets. Why should you give up? If you enjoy what you are doing there should be no reason to stop. This will also help you maintain your weight loss when you have reached your target.

One way of increasing variety in your diet is to take advantage of what foods are in season and even if you cannot grow your own, these will be the freshest, most aromatic and tastiest at the greengrocers. Also, they will have not been flown half way round the world and therefore will be the least expensive. There is something joyous about the arrival of the first runner-beans of summer simply served with sage butter, black pepper and a crisp Loire rosé, or the blackberries of early autumn picked in the late afternoon sun and eaten that evening. But really, would you want them all year round?

Hopefully, within this book, I can introduce you to some new ideas. The recipes are just some suggestions. Experiment. Experimentation can be the mother of variety in your dietary and sex life. A detailed and extensive catalogue or weekly regime would contradict the principles that are aimed at cultivating and heightening your sensual experiences and rejoicing in the joys that food, sex and life can hold.

Lastly, and unfortunately, it is the exception that proves the rule. There is but one rule in this diet. No snacks, or in other words, have nothing on the side!

Food

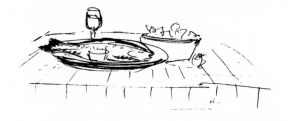

Chapter 2

Food

KNOWLEGDE

Perhaps at this stage it would be helpful to gain some basic understanding about the food we eat, why we need to eat and how our bodies use what we do eat. Food has two functions; as fuel and as building blocks for the body. As a fuel this seems straight forward, but we do not just use "unleaded" or "diesel". In fact much of what we eat can be used as fuel. Carbohydrates (or starch) are really loads of sugar molecules strung together. We digest these, breaking them back into sugar molecules, which the body burns easily. The advantage of eating starches from, for example, wheat, rice or corn, is that these energy sources are more sustained release than just eating sugar. This enables the body to use the energy rather than the more boom and bust effect of sugar, which may result in some of it ending up as fat.

Fat is a wonderful biological invention (I kid you not). It's a great way to store energy. Weight for weight there is about twice as much energy stored in fats than in carbohydrates. Imagine if there were no fat and we stored our excess energy as carbohydrate - how much heavier we would be! How big would hedgehogs have to get before their winter hibernation? This is of course a double-edged sword for those trying to lose weight since they will need to do twice as much exercise to lose the same amount. To make things worse the body makes its own short-term energy reserve which is a bit like starch and which the body uses up first before turning to the longer term fat reserves which it seems to want to hang on to for a rainy day.

Proteins are lots of amino-acid molecular building blocks stuck together. Although this sounds unnecessarily scientific the idea is simple, and like Lego (or at least the Lego of the past when there were only about twenty different sorts of bricks) there are only a certain number of different types of blocks which can be made into an infinite number if things. Digestion breaks the proteins down into these amino-acids which we absorb and build into new proteins. The instruction leaflet is DNA. But why build more, we are trying to lose weight? In fact the body is always rebuilding itself, for example replacing our skin on an almost weekly basis. This is where much of the dust in our homes comes from. Our hair and nails grow. In the same way most of our body is gradually and repeatedly replaced. Although we lose dead skin and hair, the body dislikes waste and any amino-acids left over from this *painting the Forth Railway Bridge*-like process are used as energy. The body would hate to have to use any of that valuable fat reserve unnecessarily. Damn!

The body needs other things for the process of building and maintenance. Minerals such as calcium or iron for bone and blood respectively. Sodium in salt is needed in all body fluids. Other minerals are however essential particularly for the smooth running of these processes. This is also the case for vitamins; vitamin A, for example from carrots, is needed to make the eye sensitive to light. A little cholesterol is needed too and the body will make it if required! Along with cholesterol, omega-fatty acids (predominantly from fish oils) are also important to enable the envelopes that enclose the cells of the body to work, particularly facilitating communication between the cells so that they can work in a co-ordinated way. This is most evident in the brain and that is why fish, particularly oily fish, is good for brains!

HERBS

Herbs have a central position in this diet. They are primarily used for their culinary purpose although there may just be a direct benefit that also enhances your sexual pleasures. Both herbs and spices are used in fact since the distinction and differences are difficult to draw, although herbs tend to be milder tasting and best used fresh, while spices are more pungent and are used dried.

Herbs have been used for millennia; documented accounts date back to 5000BC in China. They were extensively used by the Egyptians and the Ancient Greeks. Aristotle maintained a garden with over 300 varieties. The Romans introduced many of our herbs to this country. After the fall of the Roman Empire, much of what had been learnt was maintained by the monasteries. Later, in the seventeenth century, Culpepper popularised herbalism but also linked it with astrology. The association with the supernatural was not surprising since illness was conceptualised in terms of witchcraft, the breaking of taboos or disease-spirits.

Herbs were also grown for their beauty, for scattering to mask odorous atmospheres (before sanitation), and for witchcraft. Parsley reputably aided flight by broomstick! Herbs and spices in cooking were probably first used as preservatives, for example, rosemary, thyme and mugwort having antiseptic qualities, or were used to mask the flavour of ageing meat. In Tudor times they were used to enhance flavour and many of the dishes then resembled those of the Middle East today.

There was a decline in herbalism with the rise of synthetic medicines and a scientific understanding of the causes of illnesses, but an off-shoot (aromatherapy and a later association with massage) started at the beginning of the twentieth century. More recently, with growing disillusionment with medicines from the multinational pharmaceutical industry there has again been an increased interest in more "natural" cures, although paradoxically at the beginning of the twenty-first century these companies are scouring the flora of the world for new drugs. This book does not proffer a list of specific herbal cures for sexual ailments such as impotence, anorgasmia, premature ejaculation or lack or loss of sexual desire. Some of these appear quite unpalatable. For example, I offer but one love potion. For this you will need periwinkle, a succulent and earthworms, pounded together in a pestle and mortar and taken orally. I must admit that I do not personally recommend this and for the foreseeable future I have no intention of trying it. Of perhaps greater interest and relevance is the potential of fennel seeds for dieting. The Greek name for fennel is "marathon" which means to grow thin. Medieval monks would chew these seeds during Christian fasts to help stave off hunger.

I have tended to use herbs in large quantities in my recipes, perhaps greater than you have encountered before. This is partly to compensate for the lower quantities of fats, oils and added sugars and secondly (assuming that you are using growing herbs) they add a freshness, vitality and colour to the dish. Can herbs benefit and enhance your sexual pleasures too? Of course, a jostick smouldering in the bedroom can set the scene, relaxing and exotic; as can a bath sprinkled with rose petals, rose geranium leaves, bay leaves or lemon balm. This bath should be taken together. Also invest in some massage oil or even prepare your own. More intriguingly some herbs are attributed powers of increasing sex drive, performance, pleasure or fertility. In ancient Greece wives would welcome home returning soldiers with sage tea to encourage sexual advances although one doubts that they needed much encouragement. Anise, the basis for a number of Mediterranean liqueurs, was given to newlyweds to excite passion and beware an overdose of parsley given its libidinous powers: if it can make witches fly it may turn you or your partner into a nymphomaniac! Many spices, particularly chilli, ginger and cinnamon, are also regarded as aphrodisiacs. In the Middle Ages a drink containing nutmeg and mace was given to a bridegroom on his wedding night to increase passion. Fenugreek (used in curries) is a treatment for impotence in Chinese medicine and burdock roots (of dandelion and burdock fame) were eaten in Eastern Europe for the same reason. As an aside, willow has been used as an anti-libidinous treatment, and to ensure chastity Medieval monks would take chasteberry, otherwise known as "monks' pepper".

In addition, many herbs may reduce general health problems which can interfere with sexual performance. These conditions include high blood pressure, high cholesterol levels, diabetes and rheumatism. Garlic in particular may be helpful for the first three and sesame may reduce cholesterol. Claims are made that juniper, horseradish and liquorice will help with rheumatism although I would put no reliance on angelica to overcome one of the commonest causes of sexual under-performance, namely excess alcohol.

EATING

The recipes in the next chapter are arranged only in a vague order according to the predominant herb used. They are an eclectic group that I enjoy. There are few puddings, although I like a platter of two or three figs (fresh or dried) cut into segments or slices, a dozen almonds, a dozen chocolate coffee beans, or four squares of high quality chocolate, along with one or two other fruits, fresh, dried or glacé; sliced or segmented. This is surprisingly satisfying with coffee. With something like this it is worth making the effort, nourishing the eye as well, and presenting it on a large white plate with a sprig of mint or a light dusting of icing-sugar. Usually, however, the leisurely preparation and consumption of a single course should be sufficient. The best meals are savoured and you leave the table wanting just that little bit more (as you might in France) rather than being rushed affairs that leave you feeling gorged.

The phrase *leave the table* is also important. All too often in this country we do not pay sufficient attention to food. Sit at a table and not in front of the television. These are not *TV dinners*. Certainly pay each other attention, but also savour the food. Among the other topics of the day, pass comment or constructive criticism about the food. "If I do that again I'll write in the book that it needs more of this or that." I was always taught as a child that writing in books was tantamount to vandalism, but far from it, annotating recipe books is essential even if it is only comments like "Great; 13/08/06".

None of the recipes are complex. They rely on harmonies of a few simple flavours and the freshness and quality of the ingredients. A freshly picked green salad needs half the amount and half the complexity of a dressing that would be required for a supermarket bag of green leaves. Indeed it is surprising how little fat and salt you need with really fresh produce. At this point there needs to be a brief aside about storage. For example, tomatoes eaten straight from the vine have a sweetness that seems to be lost if you refrigerate them. I keep tomatoes on a window-sill which gets the sun. Whether the effect on sweetness is an illusion is unclear, since unrefrigerated food needs eating with much less delay. What is clear is that certain foods and drinks do taste better at room temperature rather than when icy cold; fruit, salad, cheese and red wines are among them. The reason for this is that we use our noses to taste. Our tongues have a limited repertoire of sweet, sour, bitter and salt. By smelling and via the retro-nasal passage (the connection between the back of the mouth and the nasal cavity) the aroma of food or drink gives it the rich spectrum of flavours we experience. Aromas arise from the more volatile molecules from the surface of food. Chilled foods will release fewer of these molecules and will tend therefore to taste flatter. Refrigeration, it is true, delays the more overt signs of fruit and vegetables going off and facilitates the supermarkets setting up displays of iterative colour and shape. These displays certainly stimulate acquisitional desire but it seems they may hardly enhance the end flavour.

Restaurants would like us to believe that cooking is time consuming and difficult. It is not, as I hope to prove below. As mentioned before you do need to be in the mood to cook. I also feel there needs to be a degree of thought about what is actually happening to the food during the process of cooking. This is not complicated. For instance, the browning of onions is not a charring process, you are not burning them, you are caramelising the naturally occurring sugars, almost making a toffee with the oil or butter in the pan to maximise the sweetness that is already there. When you heat protein above a certain temperature the protein molecules change shape, which is why your fish fillet curls up the instant it hits the heat. This is why you let meat such as beef "relax" before cutting into it. If you cut into it straight away it is almost like bursting a balloon and the most succulent juices are lost rather than oozing back into surface layers. You can take advantage of this. I like to put a fillet steak on a mound of spaghetti, which has no oil on it, and immediately put just one cut into the steak so that the juices spill out and soak into the pasta. Sometimes it is important not to let the proteins get too hot, for example, when making the custard for ice-cream. (As I have said there are no banned foods!) If you get it too hot you can actually see the level in the pan go down a couple of millimetres before the whole lot splits. The proteins that have been holding the oils and the water together contract and can no longer do this and the components separate. You need to start again.

This is a cautionary tale, and yes things do go wrong, but on the whole they do not. And so what if occasionally something does not work out. Is it Armageddon, losing your job or the death of a close friend? Just cook what you really want, cook with your heart and your head and have the confidence to give anything a go. Experiment. This will generate variety. Seek out recipes with novel combinations, although be wary of those that give very precise quantities. If the author needed to be so specific then it just may be one of those that is difficult to get right.

Appearance is important as already stated. Although some would argue that attractive presentation does not improve the flavour, I would argue to the contrary. I have said before that enhancement of pleasure in one modality may well increase the aesthetics in another. It would be more difficult to dispute that any of us would want to eat something that looks a complete mess. The purpose of making that little extra effort in presentation, as you might see in a restaurant, goes beyond this. It is difficult to go back and scrape out the pan in a restaurant. It is important to serve up what you are going to eat. Make up just a small amount of salad dressing and use it and if you are having bread, cut the amount you need and put the rest away before you start eating. In this way presentation not only maximises your pleasure but reduces the risk of you eating more than you had initially planned.

Lastly, it is important not to miss a meal, however busy you are. The first two meals can be very simple as outlined below, with the greatest pleasure being deferred to the evening. Weight loss should be of the order one to two pounds a week, more than this would not be sustainable. If you start missing meals there will be two consequences. The first may be that your metabolism may slow but more importantly your hunger by evening time will be so great that putting aside time to leisurely prepare and savour your evening meal will be difficult, and if you have to wait for your partner to return home, resisting snacking will become impossible.

BREAKFAST

I always begin the day with at least half a litre of dilute squash before starting on the coffee. Although it is true that instant coffee is *instant* one has to ask whether it is worth the compromise particularly since this is the last chance to avoid the dreadful stuff until returning from work.

muesli with apple

In fact any fruit except citrus or melon works well. I use standard shop bought muesli to which I have added oats in a ratio 2:1. Cut the apple into small rough cubes, on top 2-4 chopped dates and the muesli. Press down to remove excess air spaces and add milk (half-fat) to just cover the muesli and go and have your morning shower. When you come back the oats will have softened and the milk taken on a rich creaminess that is remarkably satisfying.

mixed plate

Preferably three types of fruit with either a slice of bara brith (see below), toast with crab-apple (see below) or quince jelly or really any bun or pastry you fancy.

fruit compote

Have this on its own or with muesli or part of the fruit plate. It also makes a great pudding

750g rhubarb, cut into 2-3cm lengths
juice of one orange and a few strands of thinly pared peel
1 handful of dried dates

32

1 teaspoon dried ginger
1 dessert or tablespoon (10-15g) soft brown sugar

Place the ingredients in a large pan, cover and bring to the boil. Simmer for two minutes and then let it cool in the pan without removing the lid.

kipper

Not an anaemic fillet but a gnarled and contorted whole fish. It has to be said that this in not a breakfast to conjure up before you go to work since the pungency lingers until you have cleared everything away and washed up which does not make you popular with your partner. Poached for 5 minutes in simmering water to which you have added a dash of white wine vinegar, a bay leaf and half a dozen black pepper corns and served with a few salad leaves (rocket goes very well) and a piece of bread, it is a great way to start the day.

bara brith

Traditionally, a Welsh teabread, but really a cake without fat. Rich, moist and fruity. It seems you can have your cake and eat it!

175g currants
175g sultanas
150g light Muscovado sugar
300ml strong hot tea
275g self-raising flour
1 egg, beaten

Combine the dried fruit and the sugar and soak in the tea overnight (stir well before leaving). Then simply stir in the flour and egg and pour into a greased 2lb loaf tin and bake in a preheated oven for 1¼ - 1½ hours at 150°C.

crab-apple jelly

crab apples (to make it worth doing you will need at least 2kg)
granulated sugar (the quantity depends on how much juice you get out of the apples)

Wash and halve the crab apples (there is no need to peel or core them). Place in a large pan and cover with cold water. Bring to the boil and then simmer steadily until the apples are very pulpy and the skins come away from the fruit readily. Strain through a muslin bag, preferably over night. Do not squeeze the bag, else you will get cloudy jelly. Reheat the apple juice adding one pound (450g) of sugar to every pint (500ml) of juice. Bring this slowly to the boil so that the sugar dissolves and then allow it to boil rapidly for 10 minutes, by which time setting point should have been reached. You test this with a few drops on a refrigerated saucer. If the jelly is not setting, then boil for a few minutes more. Pour into clean sterilised jars and seal.

LUNCH

I tend to eat fruit at lunchtime. I have the limited choice, as do many, of a limp sandwich, a typical canteen fry up or something that I have brought in. Few of us have enough time do more than pick up fruit. This in fact makes biological sense. We are most closely related to apes and not surprisingly our guts share close similarities. This suggests that we have evolved to eat a similar diet with a high contribution from fruit. We are fructivores, so fill up with fruit! However, do not miss out unnecessarily. If you have the opportunity to eat differently just remembering to apply the first principle of the diet, namely the pleasure to calorie ratio, by asking yourself whether the pleasure is worth the calories.

Supper

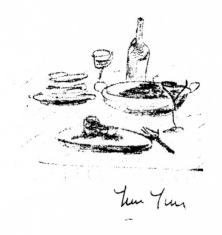

Chapter 3

SUPPER

The main meal of the day. Get yourself in the mood, think about what you are going to prepare and get your anticipatory juices going. I have arranged recipes by predominant herb since unless you are particularly well disciplined you will probably have a glut of one or other herb at any one time. For many of the final *Mixes* group you can really use any mix of herbs you fancy.

The quantities in the recipes below are appropriate for two people. I make no apology for the absence of calorie counts. Calories, or rather low calorie counts, equate with denial. These meals are about pleasure and even if exact measures of calories could be made, the more meaningful guiding principle of this book of pleasure per calorie is subjective and not open to numerical quantification.

BASIL

It is appropriate to start with the king of herbs or *Herbe Royale* as it is known in France. It takes its name from the Greek *basileus,* which means "king". Despite its esteemed position it is also an ephemeral herb, which keeps badly and should be picked and shredded as late as possible before use. In many cultures it has been associated with passion and fertility.

Its aroma is highly evocative of the Mediterranean and it is of no surprise that Culpepper wrote "it makes a man merrie and glad". This was one of the herbs I had grown in pots in preparation for our annual family holiday in Padstow. These pots of herbs were the last thing to be packed into the car, and it was the fragrance of the basil that would fill the car and generate in me a sense of impatient anticipation. There are few such simple life affirming experiences than tucking into barbecued pilchards (Cornish sardines), tomato and basil salad, a baguette and lashings of *vin rouge de table*, the accumulated heat of the day's sun radiating back from the stone walls, after a hard day on the beach.

37

The local supermarket now sells growing herbs. Along with coriander, basil is one of the two growing herbs that supermarkets do well, other herbs having been forced so much that that their flavour is but a pale shadow of homegrown. Basil needs a sunny well drained soil but unless you live in the south of the country and have a particularly sheltered spot that generates a near sub-tropical micro-climate, you need to grow this under glass and protect it from the cold. You can grow it in pots on a sunny windowsill or in a conservatory. This not only fills the atmosphere with the ambience of sunny holidays, but will help repel flies that clearly do not find the scent as attractive.

mussels provençal

1kg mussels (preferably farmed and therefore free of grit, this is different from *moules marinière* in which you sieve the cooking liquid over the mussels to serve) cleaned and bearded. Clean in cold water. A mildly abrasive kitchen sponge may be helpful, both for scrubbing the shells and also getting a good hold on the beards to pull them off. Discard any that are broken or that are open and do not shut after a brisk tap with the handle of a knife.
150g plum tomatoes (preferably skinned), diced
2 small onions or one large, finely chopped
2 cloves garlic, crushed with salt
black pepper
2 handfuls of basil leaves, coarsely chopped
1 glass (125ml) dry white wine
1 teaspoon (5ml) olive oil
1 teaspoon (5ml) butter

Sweat the onions in the oil and butter until they start to caramelise. Add the garlic and fry gently for two minutes. Add the tomato to the pan along with half the basil and the wine and turn up the heat to high. Immediately add the mussels and cover the pan, shaking occasionally over three to four minutes to allow the mussels to open. Serve in large bowls (discarding any that have not opened), spoon over the tomatoes and juices and throw on the rest of the basil.

pesto (traditional)

Although not particularly waistline friendly this is very tasty and worth having in small amounts either with pasta, grilled fish or a green salad and a robust red wine preferably outside in the evening. Shop made pesto is just not up to it once you have experienced homemade. Pounding with the pestle and mortar may give you a chance to relieve the frustrations of the day and the bonus is that pine nuts, and especially garlic, have long had reputations as aphrodisiacs in the Mediterranean and the Far East.

10-15g pine nuts, dry roast in a non-stick pan until they just start to brown
½ clove garlic, crushed with salt
1 handful of chopped basil leaves (half a supermarket pot)
¼ teaspoon black pepper
good quality olive oil
25g Parmesan cheese, grated

Crush the garlic, add the pine nuts, basil leaves and black pepper and continue to crush in a pestle and mortar (you do not want this too fine). Add the cheese and continue to pound, then add the oil a tablespoon at a time. You will be surprised how much you will need to make a thick sauce.

prawn and cashew nuts

100-150g shelled prawns (better 200-250g unshelled), best uncooked
150g spaghetti or other long pasta
4 cloves garlic, sliced ½mm to 1 mm thick
1 fresh red chilli, finely chopped
olive oil
30g cashew nuts, broken with a spoon
1 handful of basil, chopped

Put the pasta to boil according to instructions. Heat the oil gently in a pan; add the garlic and chilli so that the garlic begins to brown. Add the cashews, prawns and pepper. As the cashews begin to brown add four to six dessertspoons of the cooking liquid from the pasta, mixing and bubbling vigorously, and then add the drained pasta, which should be al dente. Turn the heat right down. Mix and cover for two minutes. Serve sprinkled with basil. No Parmesan needed.

tagliatelle and sausage

150g tagliatelle
2 high quality sausages, e.g. Merguez
½-1 chilli, chopped
1-2 sun dried tomatoes, soaked, dried off and chopped
2 cloves garlic, coarsely sliced, i.e. 1-2mm thick slices
25g smoked bacon lardons

1 small glass (125ml) red wine
1 handful of basil
Parmesan shavings, to serve
black pepper

You need to grill the sausages first, thus relieving them of much of their fat. In a small amount of olive oil sauté the bacon and garlic until they start to brown. Meanwhile cook the tagliatelle according to instructions. Add the tomato and chilli to the sauté pan. Cut the sausages into two centimetre sections and add these next, then the pepper and the red wine. (You could add a dash of balsamic vinegar too at this point to enrich the sauce.) Drain the pasta, reserving a little of the cooking liquid in case you need to add it to the pan. Combine the pasta and half the basil into the sausage mixture over a low heat. Cover for one minute and serve sprinkled with the remaining basil and Parmesan.

simple chicken

1 large onion, finely chopped
1 fresh red chilli, finely chopped
2 chicken breasts, about 125g each
175g tomatoes, chopped
100g white long-grain rice
equal quantities of white wine and water to make a volume of 175ml
large amounts of basil, equivalent to one pot from the supermarket
salt and black pepper
2 cloves garlic, finely chopped
olive oil
Parmesan shavings, to serve

Heat a little olive oil in a pan and quickly seal the chicken. Remove and put to one side whilst browning the onion in a little more olive oil. Add the chilli and garlic and continue to brown for two minutes. Now add the rice mixing round so that each grain is coated in oil. Return the chicken to the pan and add the tomatoes, the wine and water and half the basil. Bring to the boil and then simmer, covered, for 30 minutes. Do not be tempted to peek at it every five minutes; if the rice catches slightly all the better, as this crunchiness is the best bit. Once the chicken is cooked add the rest of the basil and serve with Parmesan.

stuffed peppers

2 red peppers
2 tomatoes, skinned and diced
1 handful of basil leaves, roughly chopped
1 small garlic clove, crushed
8-16 black olives, coarsely chopped
dash (at most 5ml) olive oil
dash (at most 5ml) raspberry or white wine vinegar

This really is a dish of infinite variation. Any *mediterranean* ingredient will probably work. Options may include adding a finely chopped sun dried tomato, a chilli, a couple of anchovies, a dessert spoon of white wine (instead of vinegar) or dessert spoon of rice (with an equal quantity of liquid).
Cut peppers in half, length ways. Mix the rest of the ingredients together and fill the pepper halves. Bake in a preheated oven at 200°C for 25 minutes. Serve with a green salad, crusty bread and red table wine.

pistou

This is a robust dish, to be eaten as a main course. It is yet another recipe with infinite variations. When I first wanted to make this I could find really no consensus as to method. You can add almost any other vegetable and haricot beans (cooked). It is the *aillade* that makes it. Adding chilli is unconventional and you may prefer to leave this out.

for the soup
300-350g of beans, strictly French beans but runner beans work, or a mixture, cut into 3-4cm lengths
300-350g potatoes, cut into 1 cm dice
1 largish or two small tomatoes, skinned, seeds removed and diced
1 onion, chopped
10g butter
50g spaghetti or other fine pasta, broken into 3-4 cm lengths
1 litre water
salt and pepper
and for the aillade
3 cloves garlic, crushed with salt
1 largish or two small tomatoes, skinned, cut in two and as many seeds removed as possible

1 handful of basil
10-20g Parmesan cheese, grated
1 large pinch of Maldon salt
1 fresh chilli, deseeded and chopped (optional)

First you need to start baking your tomato for the *aillade* at 180°C (it will be ready when they start to collapse in the baking dish). Meanwhile caramelise the onions with the butter in a deep pot and when golden and sticky throw in the potato, tomato (for the soup), water, and salt and pepper. The potatoes will take about fifteen minutes of simmering. After five minutes add the beans and add the pasta to allow for the appropriate cooking time.
To make the *aillade* crush the garlic in a mortar with some salt and then add the baked tomato, basil, cheese and chilli (if using) and work together with the pestle. This should have the consistency of pesto so if it is too thick add a small amount of the *pistou* liquid.
Serve in warm deep bowls with a large spoonful of the *aillade* swirled on the top. I actually like to have the mortar on the table so you can add more as you go along. Dry sherry goes very well but I think you can drink anything with this.

basil ice-cream.

300ml milk
300ml double cream
4 egg yolks
100g caster sugar
1 teaspoon (5ml) vanilla essence
a small bunch of basil leaves finely chopped

Heat the milk in a pan until it is about to boil. Meanwhile beat the egg yolks and the sugar in a bowl and then while continuing to beat slowly pour in the milk. If you just pour it all in at once you will get sweet scrambled egg in hot milk! Return the mixture to the pan and gently heat while constantly stirring until the mixture forms a thin film over the back of the wooden spoon. You are looking to make that thin watery custard that you will remember from school dinners rather than that gloopy thick stuff out of tins. If you heat it too much it will split immediately so remove it from the heat as soon as you have the appropriate consistency and let it cool. When lukewarm add the basil (if you add it to the hot mixture the basil will cook and change colour). When cold stir in the cream and the vanilla essence and chill before pouring into your ice cream maker.

CORIANDER

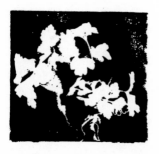

Otherwise known as *Chinese parsley*, it was used by the ancient Romans to preserve meat and has been attributed power to aid digestion, increase longevity and as an aphrodisiac. It is most associated with Indian and Chinese cookery.

Like basil it needs a sunny position although you will be hard pressed to grow it other than under glass. Small pots are ideal and you will need to sow every two to three weeks since it is the young adolescent leaves you want to cook with. Soon the leaves narrow and flower heads appear. At this point the foliage has become bitter and you may as well let it go to seed and use the dried seeds instead. Because of the need to use these young plants, buying the growing herbs from a supermarket makes sense.

tuna with hot soya sauce

2 small tuna steaks, 100g each
½ a red chilli, deseeded and chopped
4-6 cm lemon grass (you can grow your own), finely chopped
1 handful of coriander leaves, finely chopped
2 dessertspoons (20ml) soya sauce
2 dessertspoons (20ml), juice of one lime

Mix all the ingredients together and marinate tuna steaks for half an hour. Lightly oil a non-stick pan. Sear the tuna on both sides before putting half the solids from the marinade in the pan to heat these through. Ensure tuna is pink in the middle. Pour the remaining marinade over the steaks and serve with a tomato salsa and wholemeal toast.

green curry with prawns and peas

for green curry paste
½ teaspoon ground coriander
½ teaspoon ground cumin
½ teaspoon ground black pepper
coriander stalks (all the stalks from a growing supermarket pot, reserve the leaves to serve)
½ red onion
2 cloves garlic
2cm cube of ginger
1 stalk of lemon grass, finely chopped
2 green chillies
1 dessertspoon (10ml) soya sauce
1 dessertspoon (10ml), juice of half a lime
and
150g prawns
150g fresh peas (alternatively try fresh broad beans)
2 kaffia lime leaves (optional)
1 dessertspoon (10ml) soya sauce
milk from one coconut
50ml chicken stock
basil leaves (optional)
the coriander leaves
1 heaped teaspoon (5g) brown sugar
1 tablespoon (15ml) sunflower oil

Blend all the curry paste ingredients together. I use an electric hand blender and a jug, which saves faffing around with food processors. Heat the sunflower oil in a pan until hot and immediately add the curry paste and bubble for three minutes. Add prawns, peas, kaffia lime leaves, sugar, soya sauce and chicken stock and bubble for 3 minutes. Then add the basil and coconut milk and bubble for a further three minutes. Serve immediately garnished with coriander leaves on a bed of plain boiled rice and possibly with a salsa. This is easy to overcook so avoid a total cooking time of over ten minutes.

smoked haddock curry (not quite kedgeree)

1 small onion, finely chopped
1 garlic clove, finely chopped
1cm cube of ginger, finely chopped
¼ teaspoon turmeric

¼ teaspoon dried chilli flakes
½ teaspoon curry powder
½ teaspoon ground cumin
¼ teaspoon ground coriander
1 tomato, as ripe as possible, chopped
¼ red pepper, sliced
200 ml vegetable stock
125g rice
1 small cauliflower head, broken into florets
1 medium field mushroom, cut into ten
50g peas
1 handful of unsalted cashew nuts
1 handful of shelled prawns
2 eggs
150g smoked haddock, skin removed
salt and black pepper
2 handfuls of fresh coriander leaves, chopped

Don't start on the wine until you are ready to eat this one – you'll need all your faculties. There are two pans to attend to swiftly and simultaneously! Fry the onions in a little oil until they start to brown. Add the garlic, ginger, spices and seasoning and cook for two minutes, then add the tomato and a splash of water. Cook for twenty minutes before adding the haddock, pepper, and prawns and cook for a further five minutes. Meanwhile, in a shallow pan, bring the stock to the boil and add the well-rinsed rice. Then add the cauliflower, peas and mushroom and simmer covered for fifteen minutes. This should absorb all the stock. Then add the haddock mixture and 75% of the coriander. Stir in and then break the eggs on top. Cover and maintain the low heat for five minutes. Turn off the heat and leave for a further seven to ten minutes, still covered. Sprinkle with the rest of the coriander and serve.

mushroom curry

200g button mushrooms, halved
½ teaspoon coriander seeds, dry roasted and ground
½ teaspoon dried chillies, crushed
3-4 tablespoons (45-60ml) yoghurt
1 dessertspoon (10ml) tomato purée
1 small onion
1 garlic clove
1cm cube of fresh ginger
150ml water
coriander leaves

Make a paste with the onion, garlic and ginger, adding a little water if necessary. Sauté the mushrooms in the smallest amount of oil until just cooked and remove from the pan. Add a little more oil to the pan and then the onion, garlic and ginger paste and cook until it just starts to brown. Add the yoghurt, tomato purée and ground coriander and bubble for one minute before returning the mushrooms and adding water and chilli. Simmer for five minutes and serve with plain boiled rice and coriander leaves.

thai potato curry

for the paste
2cm cube of fresh ginger
2 cloves garlic
2 green chillies
1 medium sized onion
2 ripe tomatoes
1 teaspoon of coriander seeds, dry roasted and ground
1 stalk of lemon grass (optional), finely chopped
and
450g potatoes, 1cm dice
water or stock, you need to judge the amount as you add it
a couple of dashes of soya sauce
1 tablespoon (15ml) ground nut oil
1 handful of coriander leaves, coarsely chopped

Make a paste with the first seven ingredients, reserving one thinly sliced green chilli. I use an electric hand blender and a jug, which saves faffing around with food processors. The aroma that rises from the mixture is almost a meal in itself. Anticipation, like foreplay, is half the pleasure. Fry the paste until the colour starts to change. Stir continuously but do not rush to add the potatoes which then need coating with the paste. Add enough water or stock to just cover the potatoes (remember to add salt at this stage if you are using water). Cover pan and simmer until potatoes are tender. This will be about 15 to 25 minutes. Serve with a couple of dashes of soya sauce, the second chilli and the fresh coriander. You can use any vegetables that are available. A few baby sweet-corn, broccoli, green beans, mushrooms and red peppers make a nice combination.

Supper

tomato salsa

When tomatoes were first introduced to Europe and could only be afforded by the wealthy they gained a reputation (based on the rule of rarity) as fertility boosting!

3-4 tomatoes, preferably fresh from the garden, cut into 1cm dice
1 small red onion, finely sliced
1 handful of coriander, coarsely chopped
1 pinch of Maldon salt
1 dessertspoon (10ml), juice of half a lime

Mix all the ingredients together in a bowl and leave for at least half an hour at room temperature. This is great with fish and chips!

MINT

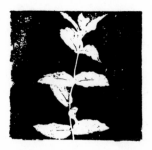

One of Britain's favourite herbs. There are various types including Bowers mint, spearmint, peppermint, eau-de-Cologne mint and apple mint to name but a few. Bowers mint is the most common mint and is that used in the mint sauce which compliments spring lamb so well. Peppermint is attributed with analgesic, antibacterial and anti-inflammatory properties. Culpepper classified it as a herb of Venus stirring up "venery and bodily lust". Shakespeare wrote of it as a Tudor *Viagra*, a stimulant for the middle-aged gentlemen. More prosaically, if also a little tangentially, sales of peppermints soared in the USA after a radio station broadcast that the hot and cold tingle could reach parts of the body that other confectionery does not.

Growing mint is no problem, indeed it is rampantly prolific and with its creeping rootstock, invasive, and usually the problem is stopping its spread. The usual advice is to plant it in a sunken container. It prefers moist soil. Spearmint will attract butterflies in to your garden.

plaice with orange and mint

2 flat fish (plaice, sole, brill or turbot), not filleted, 225g each
3 tablespoons (45ml), juice of half an orange
the other half of the orange, thinly sliced
2 teaspoons (10g) butter
1 large handful of mint leaves
salt and pepper

Grease an ovenproof dish with half of the butter. Place half the mint in the dish and lay the plaice or other flat fish on top, covering with the rest of the mint leaves. Pour over the orange juice and sprinkle with salt and pepper. Arrange the thinly sliced orange over the fish and put the half a teaspoon of butter on each fish. Cook in oven at 180°C until fish just falls off the bone (this will be about fifteen minutes). Serve using the remaining liquid as a salad dressing.

melon salad (for four to start or two as a main course)

My mint is perfectly located against a south-westerly facing wall of the house sheltered from the north and easterly winds. It however grows like a triffid and I am convinced that it has tapped its roots into the main drain. It invades the eating area on our patio so rampantly we have to do battle with it before sitting down. The mint invariably loses, but leaves behind its fresh aroma. I had not before thought of melon with mint, although it compliments cucumber so well, but this combination seems to work.

1 Charentais melon
1 orange
1 tablespoon each of mint and parsley, chopped
1 tablespoon green pumpkin seeds

and for the dressing
2 dessertspoons (20ml), juice of one lemon
2 tablespoons (30ml) olive oil
1 tablespoon (15ml) honey
salt and pepper to taste

Combine ingredients for the dressing and shake well in a small screw top jar (one of these is ideal for making dressing of any sort). Deseed and skin melon and cut into wedges or slices. Scatter the rind from the orange, the pumpkin seeds and the herbs over the melon and pour over your dressing. Best served with Palma ham and figs either fresh or dried.

yoghurt and cucumber relish

This is a cooling accompaniment to a hot curry.

1 small pot of yoghurt
½ a medium cucumber, grated
½ teaspoon salt
1 squeeze of lemon juice
1 handful of chopped mint
1 twist of black pepper
⅛ teaspoon ground cayenne

Combine all the ingredients except the cayenne, which should be sprinkled on the surface once mixed.

PARSLEY

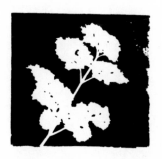

Britain's other favourite herb. There are several varieties, the most common being curly-leaved and the flatter leaf Italian parsley, which has a stronger flavour. Parsley has a long association with the Devil and witchcraft and it was believed that the long germination time was needed for the seed to travel to the Devil and back! I recently read an article which suggested soaking the seeds in boiling water before planting to hasten germination, and certainly if this did work it would add credence to the idea by reinforcing their need to be exposed to the fires of hell. Herbalists use it as a diuretic. Its claim to be an aphrodisiac may be supported by the proposition that it tones the uterus and aids lactation, suggesting that it affects the sex hormones.

Parsley is the universal garnish but is also one of France's *fines herbs* (along with chervil and tarragon) and tied in a bundle with a bay leaf and thyme sprigs a component of bouquet garni.

Parsley needs rich soil in semi-shade. It is indeed so slow to germinate, that I have often given up hope and planted another row only to be confounded the following week by flecks of green beginning to show in the first. Pick regularly and cut off the flowers for two reasons. Firstly, once it has flowered the leaves take on a bitter flavour and secondly by preventing it from flowering you can make this recalcitrant biennial last three years.

stuffed mackerel

This is a cracking way to cook mackerel, especially on a barbecue. Serve with a simple salad of tomatoes, sliced onion, coriander or basil and lemon juice or balsamic vinegar along with fresh bread and lashings of red table wine; outside in the sun, maybe after a long day on the beach. It is hot, with half a chilli per fish, so this with the parsley might get you going, a perfect end to a perfect day. Each person will require one large or two small fish which will need filleting.

per fish
½ teaspoon coriander seeds, crushed
¼ teaspoon turmeric
2 cardamom pods, seeds removed and crushed
½ a chilli, deseeded and finely chopped
1 tablespoon of finely chopped parsley
1 squeeze of lemon juice
Maldon salt and black pepper

Mix all the ingredients except the salt and pepper. Spread the mixture between the fillets and tie up with string. Sprinkle the skin with the salt and pepper. Cook on a skillet or barbecue.

moules marinière

A classic northern French dish. You could use cider instead of wine.

1kg mussels, cleaned. (Clean in cold water. A mildly abrasive kitchen sponge may be helpful, both for scrubbing the shells and also getting a good hold on the beards to pull them off. Discard any that are broken or that are open and do not shut after a brisk tap with the handle of a knife.)
15-25g butter (oil is no substitute here)
1 onion, largish, finely chopped
1-2 cloves garlic, finely chopped
150ml (1 large glass) white wine or dry cider
1 handful of chopped parsley

Sauté onions and garlic in the melted butter briefly so they become translucent, but not such that they start to brown. Add the wine and turn up the heat. When the wine is bubbling vigorously throw in the mussels and most of the parsley. Shake the pan regularly and avoid the temptation to look for three to four minutes. When all the mussels are well open transfer to serving dishes and strain the cooking liquor over. Garnish with the remaining parsley and season further with salt and pepper.

cod with cannellini beans

300g cod loin or fillet
100-150g cannellini beans, cooked weight, easiest out of a tin
1 dessertspoon capers
1 dessertspoon small chopped gherkins
a few leaves of parsley, finely chopped
1 tablespoon (15ml) mayonnaise
1 tablespoon (15ml) olive oil
a few leaves of basil, chopped
(You can make your own mayonnaise but unless you have great stamina I would suggest from personal experience that you do not use a hand whisk.)

Mix the mayonnaise, olive oil and basil and leave for the flavours to infuse. Heat the cannellini beans and mix with capers, gherkins, parsley and a little salt and pepper; keep warm while cooking the fish. Cook the fish whichever way you like, e.g. bake covered in the oven or sear.
Serve by dividing the beans between the plates. Place the fish on the beans and then spread some of the basil mayonnaise on each fish. I would recommend serving with roast garlic cloves, which are beautifully creamy, and rosemary potatoes.

spaghetti with clams and white wine

All shellfish are attributed aphrodisiac properties. Unfortunately *fruit de mer* is impractical as a regular meal. This dish however tastes quite special.

clams (cockles or even mussels) in brine from a small tin, juice reserved
1 tablespoon (15ml) olive oil
1 shallot or small onion, finely chopped
1 garlic clove, crushed
200g ripe tomatoes, chopped
2 tablespoons (30ml) white wine
150g spaghetti or other long pasta
1 handful of parsley, chopped

Make a tomato sauce by sweating onions, then adding tomato, garlic, liquid from the tin, wine and salt and pepper. Simmer for twenty minutes, meanwhile cooking the spaghetti. When the spaghetti is almost cooked add clams (or whatever) to the sauce along with the parsley. Heat through and pour over the spaghetti to serve.

walnut pesto

One of my family's favourites. Even better than the real thing and great just with pasta.

10-15g walnuts, dry roast in a non-stick pan
1 handful of parsley, broad-leaved, chopped
¼ clove garlic
25g Parmesan cheese, grated
salt and pepper as before
50/50 walnut and groundnut oil

Use the same method as before for traditional pesto, p.38.

very simple pasta

I have always found that when in a foreign city the best inexpensive restaurants are in the red light districts. This dish is derived from pasta puttanesca, which was the traditional fare of the prostitutes of Naples. Puttanesca means *prostitute style* and it certainly is a hot, spicy and exciting dish. Reputably it was placed in the windows of the bordellos to attract clients who could enter on the pretence of paying for dinner! Pasta puttanesca includes chilli and anchovies and has a cooked tomato sauce so if you want to do this start in a similar way to *spaghetti with clams and white wine* (p.51). It is fairly quick to do and it has been said to be ideal for the "working woman", although the one below is simpler and quicker and is one to do even if you are not in the mood. This is nice hot or cold and you could add chilli and anchovies to it if you like.

150g pasta shapes
1 tablespoon (15ml) olive oil
1 dessertspoon (10ml) balsamic vinegar
black pepper
1 large handful of parsley, chopped
3 sun dried tomatoes, thinly sliced
20-30 capers, well rinsed

10-15 black olives, chopped
1 garlic clove, crushed

Combine all the ingredients in a bowl, except the pasta. Mix with the drained pasta in the saucepan in which it was cooked. Serve with green salad, fresh baked crusty bread and red table wine.

parsley risotto

Risotto has a reputation as something that is difficult and labour intensive. This is a method that works well and really involves a minimum of effort. I admit that this is not a slimming dish but the portions are small and it needs a naked green salad of rocket as its only accompaniment, although a few sautéed wild mushrooms go brilliantly too. The variations are endless. You could try the two more unusual variations below as well.

1 large bunch of parsley, chopped including the stalks
½ a leek (about 50-75g), finely sliced
75g of risotto rice
225-250ml of chicken stock
25g Parmesan cheese, grated
black pepper
a very small knob of butter, 1cm cube is enough
1 dessertspoon (10ml) olive oil

You will need a pan with a lid that can go in an oven. Melt the butter and the oil and sauté the leek until it starts to brown. Now add the rice and mix around so that each grain is coated with the oil and then add 50% of the parsley (include all the stalks) and black pepper. Stir round once and add the stock. Cover the pan and then put in an oven at 150°C for twenty minutes. Then stir in the rest of the parsley and the cheese and return to the oven uncovered for fifteen minutes. Serve with lemon wedges.

cress risotto

1 large bunch of watercress (I grow land cress because like many people I have no fresh water stream running though my garden).
1 small onion, finely chopped
75g risotto rice
225-250ml chicken stock
25g Parmesan, grated
black pepper, oil and butter as before
The method is exactly the same.

vine leaf risotto

I recommend that everyone grows just one vine. Stuffed vine leaves are wonderful and the inspiration for this. If you do get grapes it is a great bonus.

10 small sweet vine leaves (July is the best time)
small bunches of dill, mint and parsley, chopped
20g pine nuts, dry roasted
75g risotto rice
225-250ml water or chicken stock
1 dessertspoon (10ml), juice of half a lemon
1 teaspoon (5g) sugar
25g Parmesan cheese, grated
oil and butter as before

The method is as before.

chicken terrine

1kg chicken, jointed, you only need the breast and wings so keep the legs for another time and use the carcass to make chicken stock. *
125g chicken liver
250ml medium to sweet white wine
1 bunch of parsley, stalks cut off and leaves finely chopped
3 cloves garlic
bouquet garni, (a bay leaf, thyme and the parsley stalks)
half a dozen black pepper corns
2 slices of smoked bacon
¼ teaspoon salt

In a small casserole place the chicken, wine, 2 cloves of garlic, bouquet garni, salt and pepper. Use kitchen foil to seal the lid as well as possible and cook in the oven at 180°C for an hour adding the liver about five to ten minutes before the end. Remove the chicken and liver and finely chop the breast meat and the liver (discard the wings). Do not use a food processor since the terrine will be too smooth. Mix the meat with the parsley. If you have one, pour the liquid from the casserole into a gravy separator, if not try to remove any of the fat from the surface with a spoon. Rub the inside of a terrine dish with the third garlic clove and line with the two bacon rashers. Place the meat and parsley mixture in the terrine and pour over the liquid from the casserole. Place greaseproof paper and then foil over the terrine and bake for a further twenty minutes. On removal place a 500g weight on the terrine as it cools. Refrigerate. Serve sliced with a green salad and brown toast.

* *To joint a bird; locate the breast bone and cut away the breast meat on one side working towards the wing joint. When you reach this, cut through it. Cut this piece in two so you have a breast and a wing. Locate, using your fingers, the joint where the leg joins the body and pull it away from the body so you can see the joint and then cut through it. Cut the leg in two at the knee joint. Do the same on the other side and you have eight joints and a carcass. It is worth making your own chicken stock with the carcass since it is easy. Place it in a pan with an onion and a carrot, both chopped in half, but leave the skin on, along with a bouquet garni, a few black pepper corns, half a teaspoon of salt and 500ml cold water. Bring to the boil and simmer for 45 minutes and then let it cool in the pan. Remove all the bits or strain. Freeze for later use.*

tomato, onion and parsley relish

To go with curry. The parsley produces a good contrast of flavours.

½ red onion, finely diced
10 cherry tomatoes, quartered
1 large handful of flat leaf parsley, chopped
½ level teaspoon salt
⅛-¼ level teaspoon cayenne pepper
½ teaspoon cumin seeds, roasted and ground
1 dessertspoon (10ml) lemon juice

Mix together and leave for half an hour.

SAGE

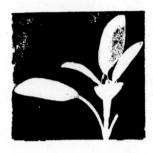

There are a number of varieties but you will only need one plant since this is a herb that, due to its strong pronounced flavour, is not that flexible. Traditionally it goes well with fatty meats such as pork, duck or goose and with offal. It goes well with beans too. Sage is said to increase libido, as are beans. So concerned about this was St Jerome that he forbade consumption of beans by nuns because of their inflammatory properties! I have included two recipes with beans so that you can test this one out. Sage has also been used by herbalists to treat colds and menopausal flushes and stimulate fertility.

Plant your specimen in a sunny spot preferably in well-drained and alkaline soil. At the end of the first year cut off the tips of the shoots and then prune annually in mid summer to promote bushy growth.

pasta with mushrooms and chestnut pesto

This meal I find is remarkably evocative of walking through a forest in early autumn as the first fallen leaves are being trodden under foot. Many of our woods still contain sweet chestnut so there is a chance here to get back to your hunter-gatherer roots and effectively collect your whole tea. This is very satisfying, although identifying your own sweet chestnuts is much easier than deciding which is edible fungi.

300g sweet chestnuts, a small cut made in each (If you don't they will explode in your oven!)
6 cloves garlic
2 handfuls of sage leaves, (30-40)
300g mixed fresh mushrooms
1-2 tablespoon (15-30ml) 50/50 groundnut/olive oil
25g Parmesan cheese, grated
salt and black pepper
150g pasta

Put the chestnuts and garlic into a preheated oven at 180°C for 25 minutes. Shell chestnuts and skin garlic. Pound the chestnuts, garlic and cheese with two thirds of the sage leaves in a mortar and season with salt and pepper. Stir in the oil to make a paste. Dry fry mushrooms throwing in the remaining sage leaves just when they are beginning to look cooked. Meanwhile cook pasta according to instructions and reserve a little of the cooking liquid. Add pesto and pasta to the mushrooms and one to two tablespoons of the cooking liquid (you may need more). Serve immediately and although this may sound clichéd, experience autumn on a plate.

runner beans and sage with prosciutto

Sage and runner beans are at their best at the same time.

250g runner beans
12 sage leaves
1 shallot sized onion
3 slices of prosciutto
2 slices from half a lemon and use the remainder for juice
1 dessertspoon (10ml) olive oil
salt and black pepper

Slice beans and very finely chop the sage and onion. Put in a baking dish with the olive oil and mix together by hand. Sprinkle with salt and pepper and place prosciutto and lemon slices on top so as to completely cover the beans and squeeze over the lemon juice. Bake at 200°C for twelve to fifteen minutes. The prosciutto becomes crispy and the beans infuse with the sage steam. Alternatively you can have this as a main meal if you roughly double the quantities. In addition slice tomatoes and throw 25g Gruyere cheese on top. Serve with fresh bread and a crisp white wine in the early autumn sun.

prosciutto and broad bean pasta

Although this sounds quite similar to the previous recipe it is in fact quite different.

4 slices of prosciutto cut into 2cm wide strips
30-40 broad beans (if you grow your own in a small garden then that's all you will get at a time. It is worth growing them just for this recipe, as fresh beans are the biz!)
6 spring onions, cut into 2cm pieces
10 sage leaves, finely chopped
1 glass (125ml) white wine
150 g pasta of your choice

Sauté the onions in a little olive oil for one to two minutes. Add prosciutto and fry for a further one to two minutes until it starts to go crispy which contrasts nicely with the silkiness of the beans. Add sage, beans, wine and black pepper. Reduce by half. Meanwhile cook pasta until al dente. Drain and add to the ham and beans. Bubble for another one to two minutes. Serve as it is; no Parmesan needed.

TARRAGON

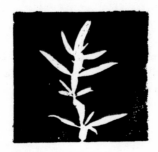

Tarragon seems quite disappointing having few therapeutic or libidinous properties. It is traditionally good with chicken and fish. Buy French tarragon and plant it in a sunny well, sheltered spot in well-drained soil. Avoid the Russian variety – it seems to lose its flavour as it grows.

poussin with tarragon

1 poussin, halved along the backbone
1 large handful of tarragon
10 cloves garlic

Supper

6 shallot-sized onions
Maldon salt and black pepper

Butter an ovenproof dish. Put each half poussin atop a heap of the tarragon and brush sparingly with olive oil. Put the garlic and onions in a bowl with a little olive oil and mix just so they get coated in oil. Toss into the dish with the poussin and liberally sprinkle with salt and pepper You want dry crispy skin when it is cooked so place in a preheated oven at 220°C for 30 minutes.

quick fish soup

Traditional French fish soup is hard work. The French go to restaurants or buy it in jars. This one is much easier.

1 onion, finely sliced
1 leek, finely sliced
2 large potatoes, cubed, about 1cm
300-350g white fish like haddock, broken into bite sized pieces
2½-3 glasses (300-375ml) dry white wine
250-500ml fish stock made up to 750ml with water
salt and pepper to taste
1 small bunch of tarragon, chopped

Fry the onions until they start to go golden and then add the leek and continue until this starts to brown as well. Add the potatoes and continue to cook for a couple of minutes before adding the wine and stock. Simmer until the potatoes start to soften and add the fish, tarragon and salt and pepper. Continue to simmer until the fish is cooked (probably only about five more minutes). Serve with grated cheddar and small cubes of toast, broken bread stick or croutons.

jugged pears in white wine

4 pears, skinned and halved
4 sprigs of tarragon
125ml white wine
125ml water
50g sugar

Put everything in a pan and poach for twenty minutes. Allow to cool and serve. You can preserve them in jars for later in the year, although the method below circumvents this laborious two-stage process. Place all the ingredients in a jar with the lid <u>placed</u> on top. This is important! If you secure the lid then you will have created a bomb! Steam must be allowed to escape! Place the jar on a tray in the cold oven and put the thermostat to 115°C and leave for 45 minutes. Turn off the oven and leave to cool in the oven for about fifteen minutes before securing the lid.

A traditional variant of this is pears in red wine. Instead of tarragon, sugar, white wine and water use red wine, a cinnamon stick, four cloves and a twist of black pepper per jar. You can get so taken away with the simplicity of this method and the idea that you are preserving a slice of summer for consumption in the long winter months that the variations are endless. Peaches work well. The fairies in *Midsummer Nights Dream* used peaches as an aphrodisiac.

peaches and apricots in white wine

4 peaches, halved
4 apricots, halved
½ a lemon, sliced
125ml white wine
125ml water
50g sugar

Use the same method as before. This is very nice with a spoon of proper vanilla ice-cream.

THYME

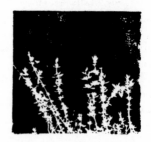

This is among the many types of perennial herb, which being evergreen can be used fresh all year round although is less plentiful in winter. Thyme likes a sunny, sheltered and well-drained position and is easy to grow from seed. It has small pinkish-white flowers that are good at attracting butterflies and bees. Angelica, chives, fennel, marjoram, rosemary and mint will all attract this magical wildlife, which will add a sense of sanctuary and peace to your garden.

Common thyme is best for cooking, being used in stuffings or as rubs for meats and mushrooms. It is a basic component of bouquet garni along with bay and parsley. I particularly like it as one of the medley of herbs on Greek salad. Lemon thyme is good with chicken and fish.

trout and thyme

2 trout
a large handful of thyme, leaves picked
¼ teaspoon salt
¼ teaspoon black pepper corns
1 tablespoon (15ml) olive oil
1 lemon
3 bay leaves, cut in half

Pound thyme, salt and pepper in a pestle and mortar and then add oil and grind further. Smear on the inside and outside of the trout and put on baking tray. Top and tail lemon so that when halved these stand stable in the baking tray. Cut slits in tops of lemons and insert 3 halved bay leaves in these. Bake at 180°C for ten to twelve minutes. Serve with boiled potatoes and a green salad. That's it, yum yum!

saffron rice

Saffron is regarded as a supreme aphrodisiac on the grounds of it rarity. In general there are two properties of food, which determine whether it has aphrodisiac qualities. The first is the law of similarities (or doctrine of signatures) by which the shape of the food dictates it effect. A typical example would be asparagus. This is more evident when you see it growing than when tied in bunches for sale. The second is the law of rarity, to which saffron remains bound. This is an aromatic rice dish that is not just to go with curry, try it with fish or chicken.

75g long grain rice
150ml hot chicken stock
10-15 saffron strands
2 spring onions, finely chopped
4 sprigs of thyme
a twist of black pepper
a few flaked or chopped almonds (optional)
10-15ml olive oil (enough to coat the rice)

Soften the spring onions in oil over a low heat. Add the rice, saffron, thyme sprigs and almonds, thoroughly coating each grain of rice with oil and heat through for two minutes. Divide between two ramekins and then pour over the chicken stock. Cover with foil and bake for 25 minutes at 150°C. Turn each ramekin out like a sandcastle.

nice potatoes

2 potatoes, cut into 1cm cubes
1 red onion, cut into quarters
thyme leaves
salt
black pepper
olive oil

I recommend either a stone baker or a large seasoned terracotta saucer. Stone bakers are available commercially and the great advantage of using these is that you can successfully roast using only a fraction of the fat or oil you would normally use. An alternative is to buy an unglazed terracotta saucer for a flowerpot. Wash and soak it thoroughly to remove any unwanted chemicals and dry it completely before seasoning it. To do this wipe a teaspoon of sunflower or groundnut oil round the inside and bake for about 15 minutes at about 120°C (wrap in foil to avoid an oily smoke haze enveloping your kitchen). No detergent should be used when washing up stoneware or unglazed terracotta.
Pound the thyme in a mortar with a large pinch of salt and pepper. Mix the potatoes, onions and thyme in a bowl with just enough oil to very lightly coat the potatoes. Bake for half an hour at 180°C.
Instead of the red onion you could do toffee onions at one end of the baking dish. This is a scrumptious combination with roast chicken. To make these;

small onions, about pickling size, you may not get them in the supermarket but I use the runts of the home-grown crop.
small knob of melted butter
1 dessertspoon (10g) sugar

Warm a bowl with boiling water and dry it thoroughly. Mix the all the ingredients together in the bowl and leave for 40-45 minutes. Then bake as above.

mushroom pasta with thyme

150-200g fresh mixed mushrooms
100-150g pasta (any shape)
4 slices pancetta, cut into 1-2cm strips
2 handfuls of thyme
salt
black pepper
1 tablespoon (15ml) olive oil

Dry fry the pancetta in a non-stick pan until crisp and put to one side. Pound the thyme leaves with salt and pepper in a mortar and add the olive oil. Spread this mixture on the mushrooms and fry in the non-stick pan to drive off some of the moisture. Meanwhile cook the pasta until al dente. Return the pancetta to the pan with the mushrooms and add a little of the cooking liquor from the pasta (one to two tablespoons). Add the drained pasta, mix together and lightly simmer for a couple of minutes and serve with a few Parmesan shavings. Sprinkle with some finely chopped parsley if you wish.

OTHERS

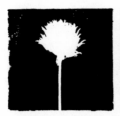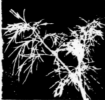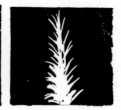

Chives, being related to onions and garlic, which are both regarded for their aphrodisiac properties, are also attributed this property by association. Chives can be used in a number of ways and go well with cheese and when used in salad dressings. They are mostly used as a garnish and that is the way I have used them here. The gazpacho below contains onion, garlic and chives so watch out. I have however included it for its wonderfully refreshing flavour.

Our first taste of any herb was probably dill, in gripe water. It has a mild aniseed taste that goes well with fish, perhaps being best known in gravlax. Fennel has a similar but stronger and more liquorice like flavour. There are in fact two distinct types of fennel. The first, Florence fennel, is an annual plant, which looks like a squat and bulbous celery. The second is a perennial plant that grows wild near the coast. It is the feathery foliage or the seeds that are used, and again great with fish. Pick a bunch on your way back from your holiday fishing trip.

Rosemary is known as the herb of remembrance, love and friendship and has a beautifully evocative fragrance of the Mediterranean. Stick some in a glass of ouzo with plenty of ice on a summer evening and you could be transported to Greece. Rosemary grows wild in warmer and drier climates than ours and therefore not surprisingly it needs sun in the summer and shelter from icy winter winds and snow. This is worth growing as it makes a handsome bush and to use the autumn prunings as a four inch deep bed on which to roast lamb is marvellous. Always use it generously and add three large sprigs to paella. The aroma that fills your kitchen will send you wild with anticipation.

I have also included rocket, partly because some regard this as a herb, partly because the Romans believed it promoted amorous desire and partly because it is wonderful as, or as part of, a green salad. If you only grow one salad leaf then let it be this one. Its peppery taste lifts a supermarket bag of green leaves.

gazpacho

This is little more than a salad smoothie. Do not be tempted to use your smoothie maker however since you will find it difficult to be free of the garlic and onion. An electric hand blender in a deep bowl works just as well and exposes you to intense aromas.

250g ripe tomatoes
1 small red onion
1 garlic clove
⅓ cucumber
1 dessertspoon (10ml) olive oil
1 dessertspoon (10ml) white wine vinegar
salt and pepper
150ml water
4-6 ice cubes
4-6 chives, chopped

and to serve
chopped pepper (red and /or green)
croutons (or something crunchy like salted pumpkin seeds)

Blend all ingredients except the water, ice cubes and chives. Stir in water and serve with a couple of ice cubes in each bowl and garnish with the chives.

pasta with prawns and peas

2 spring onions, chopped into 5mm lengths
150g cooked shelled prawns
150g fresh peas
150g pasta, twists hold the flavour well
1 glass (125ml) dry white wine
a few strands of saffron
a large handful of dill
1 dessertspoon (10ml) olive oil

Lightly fry the onion for a couple of minutes. Add the peas, saffron and prawns and cook for a couple more. Add the wine and boil vigorously until reduced by half. Then add al dente cooked pasta to the pan, mixing well, and cover. Continue to cook over a low heat for two to three minutes. Sprinkle with dill and serve outside with a very dry chilled white wine, which complements the sweetness of the peas and prawns.

salmon with fennel

A great way to serve supermarket salmon. If you are lucky enough to acquire a salmon, which is wild and very fresh, just poach it. (To poach a salmon is simple although do not be tempted to overcook, as it is easy to do. Place it in cold salted water (use one dessertspoon of salt per pint). Bring to a simmer. As soon as bubbles rise turn off the heat and let cool in the cooking liquid with the lid on. That's it!)

2 salmon fillets, 200-250g each
1 large fennel bulb or two small bulbs
1 dessertspoon fennel seeds
salt
black pepper
1 small knob of butter
olive oil to cover salmon skin
30 ml ouzo

Cut the fennel lengthways into 5mm thick slices and brown in the butter. Place in a baking dish and place the salmon on top. Lightly oil the salmon skins and sprinkle with salt, pepper and fennel seeds. Pour ouzo into the dish and bake at 200°C for fifteen to twenty minutes and serve with a green salad and bread. The juice from the baking dish may be used as the salad dressing.

rosemary potatoes

The rosemary and garlic are great together and the crispness of the potatoes and rosemary contrasts well with the soft garlic.

2 potatoes, cut into 1-2cm cubes, or chips 0.5-1cm section
8 cloves garlic, leave the skins on
salt and black pepper
rosemary chopped finely
olive oil

Just the same method as nice potatoes (p.62). Mix together all the ingredients and add just enough oil to lightly coat the contents of the bowl. Spread out in one layer on the bottom of a stone or terracotta baker and cook for half an hour at 180°C.

steak and rocket pasta

125-150g fillet steak
150g pasta of your choice
50g rocket
1 small red onion
10-15g Parmesan shavings
20-30ml olive oil
freshly ground black pepper and a generous pinch of Maldon salt
1cm cube of butter

Slice the onion thinly. Liberally season the steak. Heat a non-stick pan until very hot and add the butter. Before it has all melted (if you let it all melt much of it will burn) sear the steak. The idea is to seal it rather than cook it. Once done leave to relax while you cook the pasta. As the pasta cooks warm a large serving bowl. Thinly slice the steak and just before the pasta is done place with the onion in the bowl. Drain the pasta and add to the bowl with the olive oil. Add the rocket and mix. Serve immediately with the Parmesan and green salad dressing (p.74) on the side of the plate.

cod with red pepper

This is simple as long as you do not mind sticking your oven as high as it will go.

300g cod loin
2 red peppers

Supper

6-8 rashers of smoked streaky bacon (lardons are better however)
10ml olive oil
Maldon salt and freshly ground black pepper to season
50g rocket

Lightly grease an ovenproof dish with olive oil to stop sticking. Blanch the red peppers whole in boiling water to loosen the skin. Place the cod loin in the dish. Liberally sprinkle with salt and pepper. Cut the pepper into strips from the green stalk to where the flower was so that the pieces are triangular. These can then be arranged like a mosaic over the fish to cover it completely. Place the bacon around the fish and peppers. Bake at 230°C for ten to fifteen minutes. You need to start to blacken the pepper skins but not over cook the fish. Serve with rocket salad (the pepperiness of the rocket contrasts well with the sweetness of the peppers), French bread and a Merlot. Lovely.

MIXES

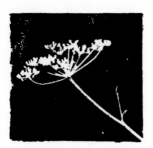

For most of these, with the exception of the Greek mushrooms, you can use any herbs that you fancy. Experiment.

vegetable soup

1 red onion, sliced
3 large carrots, chopped
2 yellow peppers
1 garlic clove, chopped
1 medium potato, chopped
1 apple, peeled, cored and chopped
1 bay leaf
1 small bunch of thyme, leaves removed
2 teaspoons of dried mixed herbs
1 knob of butter

50-75 ml milk
750-800ml vegetable stock

Bake peppers on a roasting tray in the oven at 220°C for half an hour until blistered and brown. Place in a bowl and cover with a cloth until cool enough to handle and then skin, remove seeds and chop. Melt the butter in a pan and sauté onion and garlic until soft. Add carrots, potato and apple and continue to sauté for a couple of minutes before adding the herbs and stock. Bring to the boil and simmer for twenty minutes. Then add the roasted pepper and simmer for a further fifteen minutes. Blitz with a hand blender, mix in the milk and heat through but do not boil.

greek salad

½ cucumber, peeled and cut into bite sized chunks
1 beef tomato, sliced
6-8 spring onions, chopped
10-20 black olives
50g feta cheese, cut into 1cm cubes
only one dessertspoon olive oil
salt and pepper
1 dessertspoon marjoram leaves
1 dessertspoon thyme leaves
1 dessertspoon mint, chopped
1 dessertspoon dill or fennel, chopped

Mix in a shallow bowl and leave for half an hour at room temperature for the flavours to amalgamate before serving.

basic tabouleh

125g bulghur wheat
3 tomatoes, peeled and chopped
4 spring onions, chopped
4 tablespoons parsley, chopped
4 tablespoons mint, chopped
2 dessertspoons (20ml), juice of one lemon
3 tablespoons (45ml) olive oil
salt, and black pepper

Cover bulghur wheat with cold water in a bowl. Soak for about 40 minutes or until the grains begin to soften. Combine the remaining ingredients in a serving bowl. When the wheat is soft strain though muslin or an clean linen tea-towel. Squeeze out the excess water. Mix everything and serve.

mega herb spaghetti

1 large bunch of herbs including mint, parsley and basil, chopped
grated rind of half a lemon
20 pine nuts roasted and coarsely chopped
black pepper
1-2 cloves garlic, sliced
1-2 dessertspoon (10-20ml) olive oil
150g spaghetti

Gently fry the garlic in the oil until it just starts to brown. Then add all the other ingredients (except basil if you are using which you mix in as you serve up) Add eight to ten desertspoons of the cooking liquid from the spaghetti, simmer and mix vigorously. This will produce an emulsion with the oil. When the spaghetti is al-dente, drain and add to the pan. Mix and cover for two minutes. Serve with the shredded basil, Parmesan cheese and a green salad.

roast chicken

I think the best way to eat chicken is spit roast and served with half a bottle of ice cool dry sherry as served in small bars in Seville. However, this is best consumed there and can hardly be recommended as part of a regular diet. Roast chicken is a favourite but all too often stuffed with some re-hydrated gloop, the packet for which probably has as much flavour as it's contents. This stuffed chicken however is cracking.

200g breadcrumbs
3 shallots, finely chopped
large bunches each of parsley, dill and mint
a small knob of butter or olive oil
grated rind of one lemon
1 dessertspoon (10ml) fragrant Greek honey
10 black olives, chopped
salt and black pepper

and a small to medium chicken

Sweat down shallots in the butter or oil and mix with the other ingredients. Stuff the chicken and weigh it. Roast at 180°C for twenty minutes plus twenty minutes per pound (total weight including stuffing). Serve with mixed roast vegetables (potato, onion, pepper and/or aubergine) and lightly steamed runner beans.

stuffed marrow

This is a great meal. Don't bother though unless you have seen the marrow growing and you can testify to its freshness. Serve this with steamed runner beans and baked tomatoes and this usurps cucumber sandwiches as the quintessential taste of the English summer. A whole standard sized marrow is really enough for four. If you cannot get a small one, keep the other half for the next day (cut it into four centimetre chunks and steam it for five to eight minutes as a vegetable). The following makes enough stuffing for four since eggs come in whole numbers. Freeze half of it to stuff another small marrow or even a chicken at a later date.

1 small marrow, peeled, split lengthways and seeds scooped out.
250g minced pork
150g chorizo, finely chopped if you don't have a mincer
1 slice of white bread, crumbed (it is easier to do this if you keep frozen sliced bread and crumb it while frozen on a grater)
1 tablespoon black olives, sliced
1 dessertspoon sun dried tomato paste
1 teaspoon finely grated orange peel
1 small onion, finely chopped
1 small bunch of mint, finely chopped
1 small bunch of parsley, finely chopped
1 small egg, beaten
salt and black pepper
½ teaspoon paprika
a pinch of cayenne pepper

Combine the ingredients in a bowl and bind them together with an egg. Place the mixture in the cavity of the marrow, making a sausage onto which the other half of the marrow is placed. Wrap tightly in buttered foil. Place on a baking tray in a preheated oven at 180°C for about 50 minutes (an hour if you are doing a marrow for four). The marrow should be soft when the foil is prodded.

greek mushrooms

This is enough as your main course for two with bread and the rest of the wine.

400g button mushrooms
4 shallots, chopped
4 tomatoes, skinned and chopped
4 tablespoons (60ml) white wine
¼ teaspoon ground coriander
¼ teaspoon ground black pepper
salt
2 tablespoons (30ml) tomato purée
1 sprig of thyme
1 bay leaf
1 handful of oregano, chopped
1 bunch of parsley, chopped

Fry the shallots until soft. Add tomatoes, herbs (except parsley) and spices, stirring to mix well. Add wine and mushrooms and simmer, covered, for ten minutes. Remove mushrooms to a serving dish and reduce the remaining liquid stirring in the tomato purée. Spoon over the mushrooms and sprinkle liberally with parsley. Chill and serve.

MISCELLANEOUS

BREAD

white

Making your own bread is impractical on a daily basis. It is, however, a very relaxing and satisfying pursuit that can boost your confidence as a cook, and you can experiment.

300g strong bread flower
½ sachet of bread yeast
1 teaspoon sugar
1 pinch of salt
200ml tepid (30-40°C) water

Work together with your fingers and once it becomes a dough knead it for ten to fifteen minutes. Leave in a warm place to rise for half an hour, covering

the bowl. If you use cling film, lightly oil it since this dough is tenaciously sticky. Turn out into a floured flowerpot or 2lb bread tin and leave to rise for 45 minutes, perhaps in the airing cupboard. (Remember to prepare your flowerpot by oiling it and baking it several times, wrapped in foil to avoid a oily smoke haze that will otherwise envelope your kitchen and remember not to wash it up using detergent.) Bake at 190°C for about 35 minutes. The bread is done when, if tapped on the base, it sounds hollow. Good luck!

provence bread

This is much as above but add to the dough a dessertspoon of sun dried tomato paste and a teaspoon of mixed dried herbs. Because the tomato paste has some oil in it the bread will not go stale as quickly.

focaccia

This is a flat loaf. Turn out the dough after its first rise onto a floured baking stone or tray and spread it out so that it is about two centimetres thick. Making deep indentations with you finger push in olives, basil leaves, sprigs of rosemary or caramelised onions with thyme. Brush with olive oil and liberally sprinkle with Maldon salt. Leave to rise for 45 minutes before baking at 190°C for about twenty minutes.

pizza

Something seldom found on a diet menu! The quantities above will make two bases. Turn out onto a floured work surface (I find a mixture of plain and polenta flour is best) and divide the dough in two. Roll each one out to about one centimetre thick. Place on a baking stone or tray. Freeze the second base for another day. Italian pizzas are not piled high with topping so a mixture of one finely chopped sun dried tomato with basil, pepper and a crushed garlic clove and a little olive oil is sufficient. Spread this over the base with a dozen black olives and half a dozen anchovies. Whack into an oven at 190°C for fifteen minutes and be transported to Italy as you munch through it.

herb

Using all the dough roll it out as you did for the pizza. Sprinkle the surface liberally with herbs and then roll like a Swiss roll. Cut into two-and-a-half centimetre sections that you arrange on a stoneware dish (27cm diameter) so the pieces press onto each other as the dough rises. This will give an effect similar to Chelsea buns. Brush with olive oil and a light sprinkling of salt and place in your airing cupboard to rise for about 45 minutes. Bake at 190°C for about 25-30 minutes.

grape

This is an Italian bread made to celebrate the grape harvest.

1 pizza base
300g grapes, washed and dried
25g caster sugar

Mix the sugar with the grapes so that it sticks to the residual dampness on the grapes. Arrange half the grapes on half of the base and then carefully fold over the other half of the base to make a semicircular shaped calzone. Crimp the edges together and arrange the rest of the grapes on top. You may need to push these down a little. Again let this rise for 45 minutes. Bake for 50 minutes at 190°C. Allow to cool before you cut into it, but then eat it while it is very fresh.

DRESSINGS etc.

french dressing

A small but tall screw top jar is invaluable for making up these small quantities. I think it is worth making fresh since it is never quite the same each time and adds to variety. Substituting lemon juice instead of the vinegar also provides a change.

15-20ml olive oil
10-15ml white wine vinegar
1 teaspoon smooth French mustard
¼ teaspoon each of black pepper and salt

Shake vigorously in the jar to generate an emulsion. Give another shake before pouring over the salad.

dill

This is a dressing really to go with cucumber. Before you make the dressing finely slice a cucumber (a vegetable peeler works well if you do not have a mandolin) and sprinkle with salt in a colander. Leave for half an hour to allow some of the water to be extracted from the cucumber. For the dressing;

2 tablespoons of finely chopped dill (alternatively fennel)
1 tablespoon (15ml) clear honey
4 tablespoons (60ml) white wine vinegar
1 tablespoon (15ml) water

Shake these together. Dry the cucumber with kitchen towel. Since this goes so well with salmon I would suggest arranging the cucumber around the piece of fish before pouring on the dressing.

green

Salsa verde is well worth making for a larger number of people but following the Pareto principle you can get 80% of the benefit from 20% of the effort with this one.

as for French dressing, plus
1 dessertspoon finely chopped parsley (also mint and/or basil if easily at hand)
1 dessertspoon finely chopped capers

Shake as before and leave for at least quarter of an hour before use.

rouille

This is fire! It is traditional to spread it on pieces of toasted French bread and float in fish soup. Add to almost any soup. I find it quite addictive just with toast.

a piece of dried bread soaked in water, the water then squeezed out to make a 2cm diameter ball
2-3 cloves garlic
2 fresh red chillies, chopped, at least some of the seeds removed
roughly 30ml of olive oil
salt

Crush the garlic in a mortar with the salt and then add the chillies. Work in the bread. Mix in the olive oil until the mixture has the consistency of mustard.

roast tomato

2 ripe tomatoes, skinned
½ teaspoon cayenne pepper
1-2 teaspoons cumin seeds
2 tablespoons (30ml) olive oil
1 dessertspoon (10ml), juice of half a lime
1 dessertspoon black onion seeds
1 handful of fresh coriander, chopped

Halve the tomatoes and remove as many of the seeds as you can. Divide the cayenne and cumin between the tomatoes and roast at 180°C for about half an hour or until they start to collapse. When they are warm mash up in a large mortar or bowl and mix in the oil, lime juice, onion seeds and coriander. You can use this to dress a green salad and cous-cous, which can become a meal in itself.

mint sauce

Mint sauce does not come in a jar from the supermarket. I want to weep in restaurants when I see beautiful spring lamb offered with this fluorescent green muck.

1 good handful of finely chopped mint leaves, the younger and more tender the better, and not stalks
1 heaped teaspoon (5g) sugar
1 tablespoon (15ml) boiling water
4 tablespoons (60ml) sherry vinegar

Put the sugar and mint in a small jug and add the water to dissolve the sugar. Add the vinegar, how much is really up to you.

apple sauce

1 large cooking apple, peeled, cored and sliced
2 cloves
1 teaspoon of chopped sage
1 teaspoon (5g) brown sugar
10-15g butter

There are no pans, effort or complexity with this method. Just put all the ingredients in a small buttered ovenproof dish and bake in the same oven as your meat until the apple takes on a floury consistency. At 180°C this usually takes half an hour. Mash with a fork and serve in the dish that you cooked it in.

COFFEE

You can introduce interesting variety for your evening coffee by adding a cardamom pod, a small piece of cinnamon or a little nutmeg to the cafetière. The cardamom only works if you are drinking it black, but seems to give a richer roast flavour.

Sex

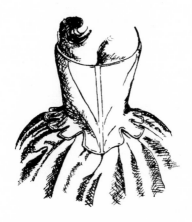

Chapter 4

SEX

If you have turned to this chapter first for a quick thrill, then you have missed the point of the book. It is evident from our discussion about mutual support, positive feedback and the spin-off benefits of exercise that sex has an important place in this diet. Most important is the proposed idea of synergistic aestheticism; a concept that by heightening the passion in one area of your life (or in one modality) you can heighten pleasure in another. Because of this, changes should be mutually reinforcing and will therefore firstly help maintain the motivation needed to see your diet to its desired end and then, secondly, help you to continue with it. Up to this point we have addressed increasing the pleasures of eating directly, and now we should turn to sex.

There are many parallels between our appetites for food and sex. It has already been mentioned that because of social constraints and taboos we exercise greater control over our primitive sex drives than our primitive hunger drives. When food is freely available these drives can run away with us. In analogous situations such as sex clubs where the sexual constraints and taboos are cast aside as a contrivance, sex becomes a quick fix but essentially empty and unsatisfying experience, rather like a hamburger and chips from a high street outlet. Pornography is another example of this fast food packaging. Artists though the ages have celebrated the sensuality of the human form. The images themselves are not degrading or exploitative. Business and the drive for profit mechanises their production and panders to our basic drives thereby potentially exploiting all of us in much the same way that the engine of intensive factory farming of food presented to us laden with fat, sugar and salt does. This is a lose-lose situation with only the manipulative profiteers winning.

Although I have emphasised the many parallels between the acts of eating and sex I do believe they should not share the same space and time. Many modern sex manuals may suggest the eating of fruit or chocolate sauce judiciously placed on your partner's erogenous zones. Although the picking of the herbs for your evening meal can set the scene and be the sensual start of an evening of sexual passion, each act should be savoured in it's own right. To mix them is to deny them the attention they respectively deserve.

There is perhaps one exception, although this involves drinking rather than eating, and this is with Champagne. I think it is a wine that travels well and travels well into the bedroom. Chill it more than recommended, and perhaps just a half bottle. After a glass each let a few drops fall onto your partner's nipples and let the chilled fizz run down their stomach, a river of ecstasy, chased by warm kisses, as the bubbly meanders on.

Herb and Sex Diet

To increase the sensuality of your sex life directly you could pursue the principles of this diet. The first two of these principles were the pleasure to calorie ratio and quality over quantity. Clearly the first does not have a direct analogy since, as is evident, making love will be calorie negative, but particularly when combined with the second it is clear that this diet is not a mandate to have as much sex as possible to burn off the fat. Quite the contrary is true. I have also discussed how this diet is a joint venture. This, however, does not mean that the moment your partner exasperates your sexual desires that you can reach for the biscuit barrel and certainly this blunt instrument should not be used as a tool of manipulation to get your own sexual way. Far from it, this is your diet and your responsibility only. The potential benefits for both of you could be quickly undermined by such narcissistic behaviour.

The first two principles were aimed at maximising your pleasure. This could be achieved by applying the second two principles of preparation and variety. Many of the Oriental books heavily emphasise time in preparation, maybe even days of massage and foreplay before intercourse. Anticipation is of the essence. Although spending hours or days in erotic preparation is impractical in our more hectic lives, phone up your partner at lunchtime and flirtatiously suggest how you want to make love to them that night but beware e-mails! Inadvertently copying suggestions for supper to a colleague or even your boss may be frowned upon but you can guarantee the same mistake describing more libidinous desires will be forwarded on to the entire mailing list. This aside, it can be a lot of fun talking about and planning an intimate evening in and considering other activities as well that can be included as part of foreplay.

Foreplay itself is an imprecise expression. Does it include widely ranging behaviours, such as the way we dress every day and use cosmetics, or is it more specific to that moment? It is a word, which although not directly addressed by the Queen in *Alice in Wonderland*, means what ever you like. What matters more than semantics, is how can we behave and what can we do that will increase the mutual pleasure and excitement of making love. The way we dress is important: the French are not only premiere gastrononauts but excel in lingerie! Shopping in an expensive lingerie boutique that is dripping with provocative lace can swell the tide of desire in both of you. Undressing too. Ask yourself, when you last undressed your partner, covering the revealed warmth with caresses? The power of kissing cannot be overestimated either, but seems an increasingly neglected expression of love as we rush into more carnal activities. Our lips are plumbed into vast areas of sensory cortex. Slow down, embrace and rediscover this intimacy. Before this, play a sport together. A psychological model called "excitation transfer" suggests that vigorous and stimulating physical exercise such as tennis can heighten the pleasure of later lovemaking and although this seems far fetched, there is evidence to support this. Alternatively just go for a walk, hand in hand. Pick the herbs for your evening meal and certainly prepare your meal together in the kitchen (only one of you needs to cook) and ensure that you eat together.

There are some foods that do heighten sexual anticipation. Although individual foods may have particular salience and associations for each of us, there is a shared unconsciousness that almost universally raises oysters as the kings of aphrodisiacs. (When you have oysters they must smell of the sea. If there are fishy then they are off.) There is always the sense of risk with oysters that probably reinforces their reputation and heightens the excitement. Oysters are in fact an acquired taste and the first couple of times that you have them you wonder what all the fuss is about. However with a glass of South Island New Zealand Sauvignon or Camel Valley Seyval Blanc, let the viscous smoothness slip through your lips and over your tongue and the taste of North Atlantic breakers explode in the back of your throat. Catch your partner's eye as you do this and the message about your desires could not be clearer if it were written in ten-foot neon above your head.

Invest in some massage oil or even prepare your own. Sensual massage takes time, so ensure that you are warm, comfortable and undisturbed. Unplug the phone. A massage is an opportunity to bring you together, learn more about each others' bodies, improve communication, gain a greater understanding of what each likes and generates a sense of anticipation that can heighten the more intimate pleasures. Start by focusing on the most tense areas and avoid the main erogenous zones. Make these "no-go" areas for a short period. This can be very arousing and indeed this avoidance of such no-go areas is a technique advocated by many sex therapists for couples to overcome anxieties that may inhibit sexual performance. Removing tension and anxiety, and relaxing, is of paramount importance. Worries distract from focusing on the pleasure that you are giving and receiving. Feeling significantly anxious makes successful and enjoyable lovemaking impossible, a phenomenon that psychologists term "reciprocal inhibition". So start slowly and be sensitive to your partner's responses and adapt your technique. Trained masseurs use a variety of moves that can be broadly divided into relaxing moves (such as stroking, circling, kneading and pressing) and stimulating moves (such as friction rubs, racking and pummelling). These are fairly self-explanatory, if not complicated. What they all have in common is touching, so try and keep in continuous contact with your partner and keep up a constant flow of movement and rhythm. You are not a professional masseur, this is not a task on which you will be appraised, so just relax yourself and concentrate on giving your partner pleasure. Equally feedback is important; let your partner know what you like and dislike and how it can be improved (firmer, lighter, slower or faster). A good way to do this is to guide your partner's hand. Swap round when you are relaxed and as your minds free of the day's woes, move onto more erogenous areas. Tease your partner; let the intensity of the touching wax and wane, and slowly move onto a more relaxed mutual exchange of erotic pleasures.

Of great importance in preparation is knowledge. Many a sexual dissatisfaction either arises or continues because of a misunderstanding or worry about the ways our bodies work. Explore and examine your own body (use a mirror) as much as that of your partner's. Even invest in a sex book. There are many informative and well-illustrated sex manuals available, although many seem to vie for attention by competing for the number of different positions they can offer.

This brings us to the other of the key principles of this diet; that is variety in itself is motivating. I decided, however, to avoid a catalogue of sexual positions and practices for several reasons. It would be too prescriptive and clinical and would not follow the spirit of the book for experimentation. Varying positions in the past were frowned upon, particularly by the Catholic Church, which accepted the law of the Stoics who in 100BC declared that couples should only use the missionary position. This probably deprived many people much pleasure and racked many others with guilt. What are regarded as normal sexual practices has fascinated, among others, a handful of academics over the last hundred years. The monumental panorama of the enormous variety of sexual behaviour was well illustrated by the studies of Havlock Ellis who published his finding in *Studies of Psychology of Sex*. In 1907 this ran to seven volumes! It seems then that variety and experimentation can go far beyond different positions.

I have already mentioned the contrast between our voyeuristic interest in the more shocking sex lives of others and our own inhibitions and reluctance to discuss our own sexual fantasies. This is a neglected area. Granted there are the stereotyped portrayals of uniforms, domination and sadomasochism and these seem well catered for by the sex industry; but less is written about what the average man or woman really thinks uncontaminated by these fast food stereotypes. Are we fearful of being labelled perverted, deviant, debased or just disgusting if we discuss these? Of course there should be no expectation that you could enact but a few of these fantasies. After all they may be unrealistic, dangerous or not fit with those of your partner's. Open, frank and consensual discussion in itself can be fun. Without it, however, you will not throw up surprises that may enable you to enjoy areas that have previously been consigned to the guilty recesses of your wildest dreams.

The seeds of these fantasies are probably formed in our adolescent sexual discoveries. This is a time we begin to find out how our bodies respond sexually. In 1966 Masters and Johnson produced what was regarded as a ground-breaking study of the human sexual response based on their laboratory studies of almost 700 individuals and couples. They described four phases; excitement, plateau, orgasm and resolution. Much of the language they used has come into common usage. Although there are indisputable differences between men and women, and functional brain scans reveal differences in the way we experience orgasm, we can still learn from ourselves. We have learnt what turns us on, what excites us and what takes us to the brink. Use this valuable knowledge. Transgress the boundaries of your own body and let your body dissolve into that of your partner's for periods, but also listen for feedback. Is what is happening for them what you could predict? Learn from the differences. We are after all individuals who seldom conform to stereotypes or textbooks.

Often lack of sexual enjoyment and satisfaction arises because of the stereotyped habits and patterns into which we are all prone to fall. To reintroduce variation into our sex lives we also perhaps need to examine what was so exciting about our first sexual encounters however innocent and tentative they were. Given the limited opportunities for intimate contacts at that age these were either clandestine encounters or risk taking encounters that stuck two metaphorical fingers up at the world if they caught you. Transgression of social rules has always excited. Social non-compliance may be why some people find public displays of affection highly erotic. Certainly making love in the open-air holds great attractions. It may be the thrill and excitement of taking this risk or is it the infectious beauty of nature that increases the pleasure? This brings us back to the idea of synergistic aesteticism. Food, after all, eaten outside tastes so much better too. There seems almost to be a reciprocity with the inspiration and awe of nature that allows ones sensuality to expand, perhaps beyond the limits of your own body. In contrast is the secret, furtive and opportunistic. The risk of discovery making the smallest noise anxiety provoking and generating an acute awareness of the pattern of your breathing that generates a focus that amplifies each millimetre of movement to an orgasm that for the briefest of moments defines your entire existence.

Let yourself go, life is full of untapped simple pleasures that are often drowned out by consumerist pressures, but which with a little attention, cultivation and effort can enrich and brighten our lives.

That said I hope, at least, that you have fun with this diet.

Herbs

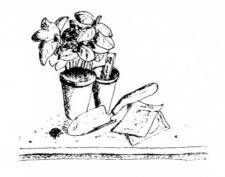

Appendix

APPENDIX

There are many pleasures in growing your own ingredients even if this are restricted to herbs. Archetypally; a warm summer evening heavy with the heady aromas of a herb garden can only amplify the pleasure of sipping a glass of crisp Sauvignion, eating and later sex. More prosaically; sitting on the ground after an hour's heavy digging in early spring, a robin singing in the nearby hedge, an earthiness on your hands and filling your nostrils can generate an almost ecstatic feeling. There is a sense of being part of the beautiful simplicity of nature and an anticipation of the first new potatoes eaten on that warm evening. In all probability the robin too is waiting with mounting anticipation to investigate your toil for any unearthed worms.

In general growing herbs is not difficult. Many are well established in this country but are not indigenous plants, having been bought here by the Romans. Remember to position your herb garden near your kitchen. The most stalwart herb lover will be reluctant to venture out to the end of the garden on a cold wet evening after a hard day at work. Below, is a simplified guide to herbs, growing, their culinary uses and their reputed properties.

Herb and Sex Diet

Name	Type	Position	Soil	Ht	Care	Companion plant	Wildlife	Culinary uses	Herbal uses	Sexual properties
Angelica	B	PS	R	2m	Plant seeds in autumn, activated by frost, transplant early spring.	-	B,Bf,O	Candied fruit, a sweetener	Anaemia, bronchitis, alcoholism	Treatment of frigidity
Basil	A	S,G	W	0.4m	From seed, tender, dislikes low temperatures.	Tomato	Insect repellent	Taste of Mediterranean	-	Passion and fertility
Bay	P, E	S,W	W, lime	13m	Often recommended to grow in tub to bring indoors in winter.	-	-	Stews, soups and stocks	Aid to digestion, baldness	-
Chives	P	S or PS	R	0.3m	Buy plant. Dies down in winter. Separate large clumps every 3-4yrs	Apple, carrots	B, Bf	Mild onion flavoured garnish	-	Aphrodisiac
Chervil	A	PS	-	0.3m	Sow directly into soil in March for summer and August for Spring	-	-	Mild aniseed, in salads and soups	-	Tudor aphrodisiac
Dill	A	S, W	W	0.6m	Sow directly into soil	-	-	Aniseed taste, good with fish	Colic	-
Coriander	A	S, G	W	0.5m	Sow directly into pot	-	-	Indian and Chinese	Digestion, longevity.	Love, Persian aphrodisiac
Fennel	P	S	W	1.6m	Buy plant or seed. Florence fennel is an annual.	-	B, Bf	Aniseed. Essential with fish	Cough medicine	-
Garlic	Bu	S, PS	W	0.3m	Plant individual cloves 5cm deep, 15cm apart in March. Lift when foliage starts to die.	-	-	Universal	Cardiovascular, ↓cholesterol, antiseptic, antibiotic.	Aphrodisiac

Herbs

						Brassica	B, Bf, O			
Hyssop	P	S	W	0.6m	Sow seeds or take cuttings.	-	B, Bf, O	A sagey/minty addition to salads	Bronchitis, catarrh.	-
Lemon grass	P	S	R	0.9m	From seed or one bulb in rooting compost will grow into clump.	-	-	Essential in Thai and Vietnamese cooking, lemon rind poor sub	Indigestion rheumatism, cramps, headache. In citronella candles	-
Lovage	P	S, PS	R	2m	Buy plant. Cut off dead stalks in winter and add fertilizer.	-	B, O	Pungent taste of giant celery. Use in soups	Indigestion and fevers.	-
Marjoram/ Oregano	P or A	S	W	varies	From seed or cutting	-	B, Bf	Marjoram is the sweetest of the oregano family. Use in greek salad.	-	-
Mint	P	S, PS	R	0.6m	Buy plant. Restrict spread by planting in sunken container.	-	B, Bf	Britain's favourite herb. Bowles mint best for cooking.	Peppermint is analgesic, antibacterial, antinflamitory.	Stimulant for middle aged gentlemen
Parsley	B	PS	R	0.2m	From seed. Pick regularly and prevent from flowering	-	-	Britain's other favourite herb. Flat leaf stronger flavour	Diuretic, increases lactation and uterine tone.	Aphrodisiac
Rosemary	P, E	S, W	W	0.5m	Propagate by cuttings or layering	-	B. Bf	An essential aromatic herb.	Analgesic, hair tonic	-

Herb and Sex Diet

Name	Type	Position	Soil	Ht	Care	Companion plant	Wildlife	Culinary uses	Herbal uses	Sexual properties
Sage	P. E.	S	W, lime	0.6m	Buy a plant. Prune in July to bush.	-	-	Good with fatty meats, offal and beans.	Colds, throat infections and menopausal flushes.	May stimulate libido and fertility.
Savory	P or A	S	W	0.3m	Two types, winter and summer. Buy in pot	Broad beans, onions	B	Peppery taste goes well with beans	-	-
Tarragon	P	S, W	W	0.5m	Get French. Buy a plant.	-	-	Transforms chicken and good with fish.	-	-
Thyme	P, E	S, W	W	0.2m	Easy to grow from seed, cuttings or layering.	-	B, Bf	In bouquet garni, good in stuffing or rubbing on meat.	Mouth washes, colds	-
Rocket	A	S	R	0.4m	Plant seed. Quickly rockets up and goes to seed therefore plant regularly.	-	-	Peppery taste	-	Romans, promoted amorous desire.
Sorrel	P	S or PS	R	0.2m	From seed, divide plants, remove flowers, harvest early (March) and late (November)	-	-	Tart flavour, use as salad leaf or with fish	-	-
Chilli	A	S, G	W	0.5	From seed. I just love growing them.	-	-	Not really a herb. Hot	Neuralgia, myalgia, colds.	Aphrodisiac

Type: A=Annual, B=Biennial, P= Perennial, E=Evergreen, Bu=Bulb.   **Soil:** W=Well drained, R=Rich moist

Position: S=Full sun, PS=Partial shade, W=Sheltered from cold wind, G=Underglass.   **Companion Plant** Plant that is protected from disease or infestation by the herb.   **Wildlife:** B=Bee, Bf=Butterfly, O=Other including hoverflies and birds

Index

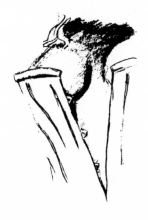

Index

Notes

Printed in the United Kingdom
by Lightning Source UK Ltd.
115572UKS00001B/169-171